DAT Prep Book

2023-2024

Comprehensive Review for Mastering Reading Comprehension, Quantitative Reasoning, Perceptual Ability, and Scientific Concepts with Full-Length Practice Tests & Detailed Answer Explanations for the Dental Admission Test

Test Treasure Publication

COPYRIGHT

Unauthorized use or duplication of this material without express and written permission from this site's owner and/or author is strictly prohibited. Excerpts and links may be used, provided that full and clear credit is given to Test Treasure Publication with appropriate and specific direction to the original content.

Trademarks

All trademarks, service marks, and trade names used within this website and Test Treasure Publication's products are proprietary to Test Treasure Publication or other respective owners that have granted Test Treasure Publication the right and license to use such intellectual property.

Disclaimer

While every effort has been made to ensure the accuracy and completeness of the information contained in our products, Test Treasure Publication assumes no responsibility for errors, omissions, or contradictory interpretation of the subject matter herein. All information is provided "as is" without warranty of any kind.

Governing Law

This website is controlled by Test Treasure Publication from our offices located in the state of California, USA. It can be accessed by most countries around the world. As each country has laws that may differ from those of California, by accessing our website, you agree that the statutes and laws of California, without regard to the conflict of laws and the United Nations Convention on the International Sales of Goods, will apply to all matters relating to the use of this website and the purchase of any products or services through this site.

CONTENTS

INTRODUCTION

Welcome to "DAT Prep Book 2023-2024" by Test Treasure Publication!

Your journey toward a rewarding career in dentistry begins here. The Dental Admission Test (DAT) Exam is a pivotal step on your path to dental school. It's not just a test; it's an opportunity to showcase your knowledge, skills, and commitment to the art and science of dentistry.

In this comprehensive guide, we've meticulously crafted a resource to empower you on your DAT preparation journey. More than just a study guide, this book is your mentor, your confidant, and your companion. We are Test Treasure Publication, and our mission is to illuminate the path to extraordinary success in the DAT Exam.

Let's embark on this enlightening and fulfilling journey together.

Understanding the Significance

The first step in your DAT journey is understanding the significance of this exam. We'll provide you with a detailed overview of the DAT's importance, the exam pattern, the administering body, time frames, and how it shapes your future as a dentist.

Navigating the Content

Inside these pages, you'll find a structured approach to mastering the DAT Exam. We've divided the book into sections that mirror the format of the actual test. From Perceptual Ability to Organic Chemistry, we've got you covered. You'll explore in-depth reviews of the essential topics, strategies for success, and, most importantly, practice questions to hone your skills.

Your DAT Roadmap

We understand that preparing for the DAT is not just about content but also about effective planning. We'll guide you through crafting study schedules, offer valuable planning advice, and address frequently asked questions to help you stay on the right track.

Test-Taking Strategies & Beyond

Your success on the DAT doesn't depend solely on your knowledge; it also relies on your test-taking strategies. We'll equip you with the tools needed to excel on test day, from effective approaches to tackling questions to techniques for managing test anxiety.

Resources Galore

In your quest to excel in the DAT Exam, it's essential to have a wide range of resources at your disposal. We've curated a list of recommended online resources and academic materials to enhance your DAT preparation.

Final Words & Beyond

As you approach the end of this book, we'll offer you final words of motivation and encouragement. Your journey to dentistry is a remarkable one, filled with challenges, growth, and untold potential.

The DAT Exam is the gateway to your dream of becoming a dentist. "DAT Prep Book 2023-2024" is your trusted companion on this journey. With our guidance and your dedication, success is within reach.

Your journey to extraordinary success begins now. Let's turn the pages and start your DAT preparation adventure. Welcome to Test Treasure Publication's "DAT Prep Book 2023-2024."

BRIEF OVERVIEW OF THE DAT EXAM AND ITS IMPORTANCE

The "Dental Admission Test (DAT) Exam 2023–2024" is a pivotal examination for aspiring dental professionals in the United States. It serves as a critical stepping stone toward achieving their dreams of entering dental schools and pursuing a career in dentistry. This comprehensive overview will provide you with insights into the exam's importance, format, and key details.

Importance:

The DAT Exam is of paramount significance for anyone seeking admission to dental schools across the nation. It is a standardized test that evaluates an applicant's academic knowledge, critical thinking skills, and overall preparedness for the rigors of dental education. A strong DAT score can be a deciding factor in securing admission to the dental school of your choice, making it an essential milestone on your path to becoming a dentist.

Exam Pattern:

The DAT Exam is meticulously designed to assess your aptitude in several key areas, including:

- **Perceptual Ability:** This section evaluates your spatial reasoning and problem-solving skills through tasks like apertures, view recognition, angle discrimination, paper folding, cube counting, and 3D form development.

- **Reading Comprehension:** You'll be tested on your ability to understand and analyze complex texts, showcasing comprehension and critical thinking skills.

- **Quantitative Reasoning:** This section involves numerical calculations, algebra, probability and statistics, geometry, and trigonometry, assessing your proficiency in mathematics.

- **Biology:** Evaluate your knowledge of cellular and molecular biology, diversity of life, the structure and functions of systems, genetics, and evolution, ecology, and behavior in the context of biological sciences.

- **General Chemistry:** Measure your understanding of states of matter, solutions, kinetics and equilibrium, atomic and molecular structure in the domain of chemistry.

- **Organic Chemistry:** This section explores chemical and physical properties of molecules, nomenclature, and functional group chemistry.

Number of Questions and Time:

The DAT Exam consists of multiple-choice questions, and the test-taker will face a total of 280 questions across the six sections. You will be allotted a time frame of approximately 5 hours to complete the exam. The division of time among sections ensures a balanced assessment of your capabilities.

Administered by:

The DAT Exam is administered by the American Dental Association (ADA). They meticulously oversee the examination process to ensure fairness, security, and the integrity of the results.

Scoring:

Scoring on the DAT Exam is crucial to your dental school application. It's assessed on a scale of 1 to 30, with a score of 18 typically considered as an average. Dental schools often consider your DAT score alongside other application components like GPA and letters of recommendation, making it a vital component of the application process.

In conclusion, the Dental Admission Test is a pivotal step in your journey to dental school. Your performance on this standardized assessment can significantly impact your chances of securing admission to your preferred dental program. Proper preparation and a thorough understanding of the exam's format and content are key to your success in the "Dental Admission Test (DAT) Exam 2023–2024."

DETAILED CONTENT REVIEW

Welcome to the heart of "DAT Prep Book 2023-2024." In this section, we embark on a comprehensive exploration of the book's content, providing you with a clear understanding of what you'll encounter within its pages. Our aim is to equip you with the knowledge, strategies, and resources needed to excel in the Dental Admission Test (DAT) Exam.

Brief Overview of the DAT Exam and Its Importance

- We begin with a detailed look at the DAT Exam itself, delving into its importance as a crucial step on your path to dental school.

- You'll gain insights into the exam's format, including the number of questions, time allocation, and scoring.

- Understand the significance of the DAT Exam in the dental school admission process and why a strong performance is essential.

Study Schedules and Planning Advice

- Crafting an effective study plan is essential, and this chapter provides you with expert advice on how to structure your DAT preparation.

- Discover tips on time management, setting goals, and maintaining motivation throughout your study journey.

- Sample study schedules and planning templates are included to help you tailor your study plan to your needs.

Frequently Asked Questions

- Get answers to common questions related to the DAT Exam. Whether you're curious about registration, test day procedures, or scoring, we've got you covered.

- Find tips and guidance on how to navigate the application process and prepare for the test day itself.

Section 1 - The Perceptual Ability

- This section covers the first part of the DAT Exam, focusing on the Perceptual Ability section.

- Explore topics such as apertures, view recognition, angle discrimination, paper folding, cube counting, and 3D form development.

- Detailed explanations and practice questions will hone your perceptual skills.

Section 2 - The Reading Comprehension

- Develop your reading comprehension skills in this section.

- We delve into strategies for understanding complex texts, summarizing key information, and answering questions effectively.

- Practice reading passages and answering questions to reinforce your comprehension skills.

Section 3 - The Quantitative Reasoning

- Master the quantitative reasoning section of the DAT Exam.

- Topics include numerical calculations, algebra, probability and statistics, geometry, and trigonometry.

- Work through a variety of math problems and sharpen your quantitative skills.

Section 4 - The Biology

- A deep dive into the biology section, covering cellular and molecular biology, diversity of life, the structure and functions of systems, genetics, and evolution, ecology, and behavior.

- Detailed content review, diagrams, and practice questions enhance your understanding of biological sciences.

Section 5 - The General Chemistry

- Focus on general chemistry topics, including states of matter, solutions, kinetics and equilibrium, and atomic and molecular structure.

- Strengthen your grasp of key chemistry concepts through explanations and problem-solving exercises.

Section 6 - The Organic Chemistry

- In this section, we explore organic chemistry topics, including chemical and physical properties of molecules, nomenclature, and functional group chemistry.

- Practice problems and explanations guide you through the intricacies of organic chemistry.

Test-Taking Strategies

- Learn valuable strategies for approaching the DAT Exam effectively. Discover techniques for time management, question analysis, and test-day preparation.

- Gain insights into tackling multiple-choice questions and optimizing your performance.

Additional Resources

- Explore a curated list of recommended online resources and academic materials to further enhance your DAT preparation.

- Find out where to access supplementary study materials and practice tests to complement your study plan.

Final Words and Motivation

- Conclude your journey with a dose of motivation and encouragement.

- Inspirational insights and words of encouragement remind you of the importance of your goals and aspirations.

Two Full-Length Practice Tests

- Put your knowledge and skills to the test with two full-length practice exams.

- Each practice test consists of 100 questions, mirroring the DAT Exam format, and includes detailed answer explanations.

This "Detailed Content Review" provides a roadmap for your journey through "DAT Prep Book 2023-2024." It is structured to equip you with the knowledge, skills, and confidence needed to excel in the DAT Exam and make significant strides toward your dream of a successful dental career. Each chapter is carefully designed to cater to the specific needs and challenges you may encounter on your DAT preparation journey.

Now, let's begin your educational adventure and work together to achieve extraordinary success in the world of dentistry.

STUDY SCHEDULES AND PLANNING ADVICE

Your journey toward acing the Dental Admission Test (DAT) Exam begins with effective study planning. In this chapter, we'll explore the vital aspects of creating a study schedule that suits your needs and offer advice on how to stay on track and motivated throughout your preparation.

Crafting Your Study Plan

- The first step to DAT success is creating a well-structured study plan. We'll guide you through the process of crafting a personalized plan tailored to your unique situation.

- Understand the importance of setting realistic goals and milestones to monitor your progress effectively.

Time Management Strategies

- Efficient time management is the key to productive study sessions. Learn strategies for allocating your time wisely, maximizing your study hours, and balancing your academic and personal life.

- Discover the power of time-blocking and setting priorities to make the most of each study session.

Setting Achievable Goals

- Goal setting is crucial for motivation and focus. We'll help you set clear, achievable goals for your DAT preparation, making it easier to track your progress.

- Learn how to break down your goals into manageable tasks, ensuring a sense of accomplishment along the way.

Staying Motivated

- Maintaining motivation throughout your DAT preparation can be challenging, but it's essential for success. We'll provide tips on staying inspired and enthusiastic about your study journey.

- Explore strategies for overcoming common motivational obstacles and boosting your study morale.

Sample Study Schedules

- Sometimes, seeing is believing. We'll present sample study schedules tailored to different timelines and intensities.

- These schedules can serve as templates to help you structure your study plan effectively, whether you have several months or just a few weeks to prepare.

Tracking Your Progress

- Regularly monitoring your progress is essential. Learn how to keep track of your achievements, identify areas of improvement, and make necessary adjustments to your study plan.

- Discover tools and techniques for maintaining an organized record of your DAT preparation journey.

Test Day Preparation

- Your study schedule should also include strategies for preparing for the actual test day. Find advice on what to do in the final days leading up to the DAT Exam.

- From ensuring you have the right materials to tips for a stress-free test day, we've got you covered.

Adapting Your Plan

- Flexibility is key in any study plan. Learn how to adapt your schedule and goals as you progress and encounter unexpected challenges.

- We'll provide guidance on staying nimble and making changes when needed without sacrificing your overall plan.

In this chapter, we empower you to take control of your DAT preparation by crafting a study schedule that fits your lifestyle and goals. With effective time management, achievable objectives, and motivation strategies, you'll be well-prepared to tackle the DAT Exam with confidence.

FREQUENTLY ASKED QUESTIONS

As you embark on your journey to conquer the Dental Admission Test (DAT) Exam, you may encounter various questions and uncertainties along the way. This chapter is dedicated to addressing the most common questions that DAT aspirants often have, providing you with clear and concise answers to ensure a smooth and informed preparation process.

Question 1: What is the DAT Exam, and why is it important for dental school admission?

- The DAT Exam, or Dental Admission Test, is a standardized examination used by dental schools in the United States to assess the academic readiness of applicants.

- Learn about the critical role the DAT Exam plays in the dental school admission process and why a strong performance is essential for aspiring dentists.

Question 2: When and where is the DAT Exam administered?

- Discover information about the test's administration dates and locations, ensuring you have all the details you need to plan your test day effectively.

Question 3: How is the DAT Exam structured?

- Get a comprehensive overview of the DAT Exam's structure, including the number of sections, types of questions, and time allocations for each section.

Question 4: What are the eligibility requirements to take the DAT Exam?

- Understand the prerequisites and qualifications necessary to register for the DAT Exam, ensuring you meet the criteria for test-takers.

Question 5: How do I register for the DAT Exam, and what is the registration process like?

- Step-by-step guidance on the DAT Exam registration process, including creating a DAT account, selecting test dates, and completing your registration.

Question 6: How is the DAT Exam scored, and what is considered a competitive score?

- Learn about the scoring system used for the DAT Exam and what scores are typically considered competitive for dental school admission.

Question 7: What is the best way to prepare for the DAT Exam?

- Explore effective strategies for DAT preparation, including the use of study guides, practice tests, and other resources.

- Find out how to create a study schedule tailored to your needs and goals.

Question 8: Can I retake the DAT Exam if I'm not satisfied with my score?

- Understand the DAT Exam retake policy and the implications of taking the exam multiple times.

- Learn how dental schools consider multiple scores in the admission process.

Question 9: What should I expect on the day of the DAT Exam, and what should I bring with me?

- Detailed guidance on test day procedures, including what to expect, what to bring, and how to ensure a stress-free testing experience.

Question 10: How can I request accommodations for the DAT Exam if I have a disability or medical condition?

- Information on the process for requesting accommodations, ensuring that all test-takers have equal opportunities to excel in the DAT Exam.

Question 11: How are DAT scores used in the dental school admission process?

- Understand how dental schools evaluate DAT scores in the context of your overall application.

- Learn how to highlight your DAT achievements in your dental school application.

Question 12: What resources are available for DAT preparation beyond this book?

- Explore a list of recommended online resources and academic materials to supplement your DAT preparation.

- Find additional sources of support and information to enhance your study plan.

This chapter is designed to equip you with answers to the most pressing questions you may have about the DAT Exam. With clear and concise responses, you'll have the knowledge and confidence to navigate your DAT preparation journey successfully.

Section 1: The Perceptual Ability

Apertures

Come on, buckle up! We're about to embark on a mind-blowing journey of self-discovery. Each page in this guide is like a door waiting to be opened, revealing a whole new world of knowledge and tricks to ace those pesky exams.

Our adventure begins with the Introduction. Think of it like the foundation of a kick-ass building. It welcomes us into the test, shows us the ropes, and gives us a map to navigate through the upcoming chapters. We gotta have our feet on solid ground if we wanna dive deep into the depths of this exam.

Next up, we stumble upon the Verbal Reasoning zone. This is where we sharpen our language skills, my friend. We gotta learn how to decode complicated passages, spot key info, and draw some serious conclusions. It's not just about knowing fancy words or grammar rules. No, siree! This is where we learn to connect our brain's horsepower with our linguistic finesse, so we can uncover the hidden gems hidden behind every single word.

Now, hold on tight 'cause we're about to jump into the Quantitative Reasoning rabbit hole. This is the land of numbers, equations, and math wizardry. We're gonna unravel the mysteries of algebra, geometry, and all those crazy mathematical operations. Trust me, it's gonna get a bit wild. But once we master the art of manipulating data, interpreting graphs, and solving mind-bending problems, we'll be ready to conquer any quantitative challenge that comes our way.

Brace yourself for the Natural Sciences rollercoaster. Once we step through this gateway, we'll dive headfirst into the captivating world of biology, chemistry, and all things science. We're gonna study the building blocks of life, the chemical reactions shaping our environment, and the laws governing this wild, wild world. This is the secret kingdom of science, my friend, and with this knowledge, we'll have the power to dominate this exam.

Alright, last but not least, we're gonna tackle the Perceptual Ability. It's like a hidden treasure chest filled with visual perception, cognitive skills, and spatial reasoning. We're gonna train our eyes to observe, compare, and manipulate some seriously mind-boggling visual patterns. It's not gonna be easy, my friend, but we're gonna learn to think outside the box, follow the hidden clues, and outsmart our senses. By the end of it, we'll be master wizards of perception, ready to tackle any challenge thrown at us.

But wait, there's more! This journey isn't just about acing some exam. No, no. It's also about growing as individuals. We're gonna gain some serious self-awareness, resilience, and personal growth. We're gonna transform from mere test-takers to badass scholars, from seekers to creators.

So, my friend, join us on this incredible adventure. Together, we'll unlock the true power of these apertures. They'll light up our path to extraordinary success. Step up and let's rock this exam.

View Recognition

Hey there! So, you know how we're all trying to kick some major butt at the DAT, right? Well, there's this super important thing called view recognition that we gotta get on board with. And let me tell you, it's not just about acing the exam.

This skill can seriously enrich our lives by helping us become super keen observers and perceptive beings. I mean, we're talking about unlocking a whole new world filled with mind-blowing wonders and mysteries just waiting to be discovered!

Alright, so step 1 on this wild journey is all about sharpening our senses, my friend. We gotta train ourselves to be top-notch observers of the world around us. You know, like when we're walking down the street or chilling in a park, we need to supercharge our awareness and start seeing everything in a whole new light. It's like going from plain ol' black and white to full-on technicolor, you feel me? By honing our eyes, ears, and minds to catch all those subtle details in our surroundings, we'll be uncovering a goldmine of hidden insights.

Now, here's step 2, and it's a real game-changer. We gotta embrace curiosity and wonder like it's our job, my friend. Instead of just glancing at stuff, let's take a moment to really stop and soak in all the awe-inspiring intricacies that surround us. Like seriously, have you ever just sat there and marveled at the stroke of colors in a stunning sunset or the vibrant chaos of a bustling cityscape? Our curiosity is gonna guide us to a deeper understanding and appreciation of this whole crazy world we're living in.

Step 3 is where things get really interesting, my friend. We're gonna dive headfirst into the realm of the unnoticed. You know how sometimes the most mind-blowing views are hiding in plain sight? It's like this secret world that's just waiting for us to discover it. You've got the moss-covered brick walls in those ancient alleyways, the way sunlight filters through leaves and creates dazzling, playful patterns, and the utterly mesmerizing dance of reflections on a body of water — these are the kind of hidden gems that have the power to ignite our souls and transform how we see the world.

Okay, now that our senses are on point, our curiosity is running wild, and we're noticing things that would make Sherlock Holmes proud, it's time for step 4.

We need to learn how to capture the essence of all these mind-blowing views we encounter. Whether it's through sketches, snagging some sweet photographs, or just etching them into our memory banks, we gotta make sure we preserve the beauty and depth of our experiences. Trust me, it's gonna create a visual library that not only shows how much we've grown but also becomes our little wellspring of inspiration for all the amazing things we'll do in the future.

Alright, my friend, we're on to step 5. This is where the magic happens. We're gonna take all these mad skills we've been developing and apply them to the DAT like pros. I'm talking about becoming visual geniuses who can observe, analyze, and put together complex visual info like nobody's business. Yeah, sure, it's super important for the perceptual ability section of the exam, but here's the kicker – it's also gonna rock our future careers in dentistry. With the power of view recognition in our back pockets, we'll be lightyears ahead of the game, both in the exam room and out in the real world.

Now, step 6 is where things get all sentimental and stuff. View recognition isn't just some one-and-done thing we use for the DAT. Nah, my friend, this is a lifelong journey that lets us keep exploring and appreciating the world around us. So, as we wrap up this chapter in our epic DAT prep, let's remember that view recognition is all about forever changing how we see and understand things. Who knows, maybe we'll stumble upon extraordinary views in the most ordinary places – and that's what makes this whole journey so darn beautiful.

Hey, by the way, over at Test Treasure Publication, they're all about the art of view recognition. They're totally committed to helping us embrace this whole new way of looking at the world. So let's join forces and embark on a journey that's gonna take us way beyond the ordinary. That's right, my friend – we're gonna ignite our passion for learning and slay the game with extraordinary success.

Angle Discrimination

Hey there! Want to dive into the fascinating world of angle discrimination with me? Buckle up, because we're about to take a journey through its rich historical timeline. From ancient civilizations to modern developments, we'll uncover the significance of this concept and its impact on various fields of study.

So first off, let's head to ancient Egypt, the land of golden sands and towering pyramids. These magnificent structures aren't just for show - they actually showcase the Egyptians' advanced understanding of geometry. Hieroglyphs etched onto the walls reveal the use of angle measurements in the construction process. Talk about early genius, right?

Next stop: ancient Greece, the birthplace of geometry itself. Here, we meet Thales of Miletus, a philosopher-mathematician who's often hailed as the pioneer of angle discrimination. He was obsessed with triangles and circles, delving into their mathematical properties and setting the stage for future angle explorations. Thales' work even laid the foundation for Euclid's famous treatise, "Elements," which went deep into the intricate world of angles.

Let's fast-forward to the Islamic Golden Age, a period of incredible intellectual and scientific advancements. This is where we encounter brilliant scholars like Al-Khwarizmi, Al-Kindi, and Al-Biruni, who made groundbreaking contributions to angle discrimination and trigonometry. Their mathematical treatises spread far and wide, thanks to translations, and trigonometry got a major boost with the development of sine and cosine functions. Talk about revolutionizing angle measurement!

Now, let's step into the Renaissance, a time of art, science, and profound human curiosity. Here, geniuses like Leonardo da Vinci and Johannes Kepler celebrated the beauty of angles. Da Vinci, the ultimate observer of the natural world, highlighted the importance of angles in capturing perspective and proportion in his art. Meanwhile, Kepler's astronomical discoveries revealed the significance of angles in celestial movements. These guys knew how to appreciate angles in their work!

And finally, in the modern era, angle discrimination has found a home in numerous disciplines. Think architecture, engineering, physics, computer science - you name it! We've got some fancy precision instruments like the theodolite and laser technology that help us measure and calculate angles with jaw-dropping accuracy. Angle discrimination has become a crucial aspect of professions like surveying, navigation, graphic design, animation, and it even spills over into artificial intelligence and robotics. The possibilities are mind-boggling!

So, let's unlock the secrets of this ancient knowledge together and embark on an illuminating journey. Test Treasure Publication has got your back with comprehensive study guides, interactive exercises, and real-world applications. We're here to equip you with all the tools you need to conquer angle discrimination and take your learning to a whole new level. So buckle up and let's navigate this intricate labyrinth of angles, uncovering the hidden treasures that lie within. Let's do this!

Paper Folding

Prepare yourself for a wild ride, folks, because we're about to delve into the fascinating world of exam prep. And guess what? We're not talking about your typical study techniques. No, no. We're diving headfirst into the art of paper folding. Sound crazy? Well, hold onto your hats because this is going to blow your mind.

Now, you might be wondering what the heck paper folding, or origami as the fancy folks call it, has to do with acing exams. Well, my friends, let me tell you: origami is more than just a way to pass the time or make pretty decorations. It's a whole new way of thinking. It taps into our creative side and gets those critical thinking skills firing on all cylinders.

Origami has been around for centuries, starting off as a spiritual practice in ancient rituals and ceremonies. But over time, it became a popular hobby and a form of self-expression. And let me tell you, there's something magical about taking a plain ol' sheet of paper and transforming it into a work of art.

But here's the real kicker—the reason why origami is the secret weapon in the exam-prep arsenal. It's all about how it shapes our minds, just like those intricate folds shape the paper. When we engage in the delicate process of folding, we're training our brains to think critically, analyze patterns, and see things from different angles.

Think about it. When we navigate the twists and turns of origami, we're actually sharpening our problem-solving skills and building up our spatial awareness. That spatial stuff is key in subjects like geometry and physics. So, you see, origami is more than just a crafty pastime. It's an educational powerhouse.

But hold on, we're just getting started. Origami doesn't stop at STEM subjects. Oh no, my friends. It's got tricks up its sleeve that'll revolutionize how you approach those pesky verbal and written exams. You see, origami is all about delving into your creative side and thinking outside the box.

When we transform that flat piece of paper into a three-dimensional masterpiece, something magical happens. It unlocks our imagination and helps us come up with innovative ways to tackle problems and write killer essays. It's like a creativity boost in a box. Or, well, on a piece of paper.

So, are you ready for the journey of a lifetime? Buckle up because we're about to embark on an adventure that will take you beyond ordinary learning. We'll explore the wonders of paper folding, uncovering its hidden secrets, and tapping into the extraordinary power it holds. Get ready to unleash your intellectual prowess and let your creative side soar. Welcome to the mesmerizing world of origami, where the folds of possibility are endless.

Cube Counting

Alright, folks, we're diving into the realm of cube counting. Get ready for a challenge that requires all your mental acuity and spatial intelligence. We'll be mentally manipulating three-dimensional objects, envisioning them from different perspectives, and counting the visible cubes. It's all about having that keen eye for detail.

When you start counting, you'll be faced with all kinds of arrangements and orientations. Cubes will be placed super close together, maybe even overlapping or hiding behind other cubes. Your job is to decipher these formations like a pro and spot the cubes that are exposed to your line of sight.

Now, what's beautiful about cube counting is how it really tests your visual skills and gets your spatial intelligence fired up. You're gonna analyze each figure from all angles, thinking about what's visible and what's hidden. It's like mentally taking apart these complex structures and figuring out how many cubes you can really see.

To really master cube counting, you gotta come up with a strategy. Take your time and break down each figure systematically. Picture it in your mind, identify the individual cubes, and keep track of your count. Trust me, you gotta have the patience and attention to detail for this stuff. Missing even one cube could mean getting the answer wrong.

But here's the thing, cube counting is not just about being a counting pro. It's about your ability to see and interpret spatial relationships. It makes you think critically and visually, and gives you a deep understanding of three-dimensional geometry. And hey, these skills don't just stay within cube counting. They'll serve you well in other walks of life too.

That's why Test Treasure Publication is here for you. We've got all the study materials and practice questions you need to conquer the cube counting section of the DAT exam. We'll provide in-depth explanations, step-by-step guides, and expert tips to help you navigate this tricky subject.

So, let's embark on this cube counting adventure together. It'll not only boost your DAT prep, but also sharpen your spatial reasoning skills. Let Test Treasure Publication light your way to mastery and guide you towards amazing success.

3D Form Development

Alright, folks, let's take a trip back in time. Picture this: our ancestors, way back when, were just getting curious. They had this itch to create, to make things with their own two hands. So, armed with nothing but their imagination and whatever materials they could get their hands on, they started shaping clay. Sculpting it into vessels, statues, and tools. It's like they were breathing life into these things, giving them purpose, you know?

Fast forward a bit and we find ourselves right smack in the middle of the Renaissance. Now, this was a time when art and science really hit their peak. You had the big names - Leonardo da Vinci, Michelangelo, Raphael - these guys were true visionaries. They were all about studying the human body, dissecting it, and then capturing every little detail in their paintings and sculptures. Their work was like a precise and perfect representation of the three-dimensional world, merging art and science like never before.

But the fun doesn't stop there. The industrial revolution comes along and suddenly everything changes. With new advancements in mechanical engineering and manufacturing, people start dreaming up all sorts of crazy structures. I'm talking huge skyscrapers that scrape the sky, and delicate bridges that seem to defy gravity. It's like they took the idea of 3D design and ran with it, pushing the boundaries of what was possible.

And then the 20th century comes crashing in with its technological boom. All this fancy stuff starts happening - rapid prototyping, computer-aided design, and additive manufacturing. These guys invented 3D printers, for crying out loud! That's like something out of a sci-fi movie. Now, dreamers and inventors can take their wild ideas and actually turn them into real, tangible things.

Nowadays, 3D design is everywhere. You can't escape it. In animation, those beloved characters you see on the big screen - yep, they're brought to life through 3D wizardry. And in the medical field, they're using amazing 3D imaging and printing to take patient care to a whole new level. It's like technology and creativity are holding hands and leading us into the future.

So, here in this book, we're going on the adventure of a lifetime. We're diving headfirst into the world of 3D form development, exploring its history, the technical stuff, and even practical ways it's being used today. Get ready to uncover the secrets and mysteries of this mind-blowing art and science. It's a journey where the past meets the present, and together, they shape a future that's only limited by our own imagination. Can you dig it?

SECTION 2: THE READING COMPREHENSION

Comprehension Skills

In our study guides, we don't settle for just scratching the surface of concepts. We dive deep into the guts of each subject, peeling back the layers to reveal the intricate details. We don't just throw complex theories and principles at you - that's no fun. We break them down into bite-sized pieces, like your mom cutting up your steak so you don't choke on it. And to bring the content to life, we sprinkle in real-life examples that light up your brain like a fireworks show.

It's not enough for us to simply understand the material - that's like saying you've learned to swim by standing on the beach and watching others splash around. We want you to be able to take that knowledge and apply it like a magic trick, in any situation. That's why we pack our study materials with all sorts of practice questions and exercises that make you think. We want you to chew on the knowledge, flip it upside down, and analyze it from all angles. It's like a mental gymnastics workout that builds your analytical muscles and makes you question everything, even your own name.

And hey, comprehension isn't just about reading. We get that. That's why we throw in some nifty tips and techniques to help you read faster and focus better. It's like X-ray vision for your eyes, helping you skim through passages like a speed reader on steroids. You'll be able to extract the juiciest ideas from any text, no matter how dense or boring it may seem. We'll hold your hand and guide you through the treacherous waters of challenging texts, so you can confidently tackle any exam question that's thrown at you.

But wait, there's more! We know that visuals are just as important as words. It's like trying to understand a superhero movie without the cool special effects. That's why we teach you how to interpret and analyze graphs, charts, and diagrams. We want you to be able to look at those squiggly lines and dots and go "Aha! I get it now!" It's like uncovering hidden treasures and uncovering the secrets of the universe.

And if that's not enough, we've got online resources that are like a party for your brain. You get to watch videos, animations, and do interactive quizzes - it's like learning on steroids. We take your comprehension skills to the next level - all while you're chilling in your pajamas, sipping hot cocoa.

But listen, it's not just about passing exams. That's like saying winning a soccer game is all about scoring goals. We want you to really understand and internalize the stuff you're learning. We want you to be a master of your own education, ready to take on whatever life throws your way. You've got potential, my friend, and we're here to help you unlock it, one comprehension at a time. Are you ready to embark on this epic journey of knowledge? Let's do this - together.

Critical Thinking Skills

So, let me tell you about the world of standardized tests. It's a real whirlwind of exams and scores, and if you want to go from average to exceptional, you gotta have a secret weapon. And that secret weapon is critical thinking. Yeah, it's not just some fancy buzzword, it's the key to unlocking your highest score.

You see, our study materials are like wizards of the mind. We go beyond boring facts and figures and dive deep into the art of thinking critically. We give you all the tools and tricks you need to tackle those complex problems like a pro.

But it all starts with a mindset, my friend. The first step is realizing that no question or problem is too big to handle. Seriously, don't be intimidated! We encourage you to keep an open mind and explore different perspectives. It's like looking at a diamond from all angles. By embracing diverse viewpoints, you'll be able to crack those tough exam questions wide open and surprise yourself with some seriously innovative solutions.

And that's not all. Our study materials are all about sharpening your analytical thinking skills. We'll teach you how to spot patterns, make connections, and dig deep into those underlying themes. Listen, evidence-based reasoning is the name of the game. We'll show you how to dissect arguments, evaluate your sources, and draw unbiased conclusions. It's like being Sherlock Holmes, only with a calculator.

But hey, we're not done yet. Critical thinking is also about becoming the master of problem-solving. Our study guides give you a step-by-step roadmap to tackle even the trickiest problems. We'll break 'em down into bite-sized pieces, making it easier for you to understand what's really going on. And guess what? We're all about encouraging you to think outside the box. Think of us as your personal cheerleaders, raising you up to conquer those seemingly impossible obstacles.

Oh, and the fun doesn't stop there. We've got critical thinking exercises sprinkled throughout our study materials. It's like a real-life test simulation, putting your newfound skills to the test under pressure. It's like jumping into the deep end of the pool, but don't worry, we've got your back. By practicing these exercises, you'll become a critical thinking champ. It'll come as naturally to you as breathing, no more forced effort required.

But wait, there's more. We're not just all about the study materials. At Test Treasure Publication, we believe in building a community. We want you to connect with other students, share ideas, and grow together. We've got online forums, study groups, and even mentorship programs. We're creating a place where intellectual curiosity thrives and where budding intellectuals can spread their wings.

So, in a nutshell, Test Treasure Publication knows the importance of critical thinking. We don't just say it, we live it. We've got the whole package to help you develop and refine your critical thinking skills. With us by your side, you'll be able to conquer those challenging questions, analyze complex problems, and come up with innovative solutions. We're here to instill a passion for critical thinking in you. So come join us on this enlightening journey. Together, let's make critical thinking your guiding light to extraordinary success.

Section 3: The Quantitative Reasoning

Numerical Calculations

Let me take you on a voyage, my friend, to where it all started - ancient Mesopotamia. Picture this: a world where numbers were just beginning to emerge, where the Sumerians pushed the boundaries and created a whole new system around 3000 BCE. They were the pioneers, my friend. They came up with these symbols to represent quantities, and little did they know, they were laying the foundation for future civilizations to build upon.

As we sail through time, we stumble upon the Egyptians - the ones who truly revolutionized arithmetic. Can you imagine? They understood fractions! They developed decimal notation! These guys were game-changers, my friend. The advancements they made paved the way for all those complex mathematical calculations that would come along in the centuries to follow.

Ah, but the sweet aroma of ancient Greece awaits us, my friend. These thinkers were the real deal. Pythagoras, Euclid, and Archimedes - their names hold weight. Pythagoras and his famous theorem about right-angled triangles? Oh, it was a paradigm-shifter! And Euclid? His work "Elements" laid down the groundwork for all that deductive reasoning stuff, transforming geometry into a beautiful tapestry of proofs and theorems. And then there's Archimedes, a true legend in the mathematical realm. That guy, my friend, made incredible contributions to the understanding of pi, areas, and volumes. It blows my mind.

Fast forward to Renaissance Europe, my friend. This is where things start to get real juicy. Leonardo da Vinci, Johannes Kepler, Galileo Galilei - these guys all had that mathematical prowess flowing through their veins. Da Vinci's calculations and geometric patterns? They were the stuff of art, engineering, and scientific research. Kepler's model of planetary motion brought a whole new level of elegance to the cosmos. And what about Galileo? His experiments and calculations paved the way for the scientific method, forever changing the game. Can you believe it?

And then, my friend, the modern era hits. Computers come onto the scene, and boy, did they shake things up. With programming and algorithms, complex computational problems became manageable tasks. The digital revolution gave us simulations, predictive models, data analysis, and optimization. It was like a whole new world opened up to us, my friend.

So, where does that leave us now? In awe, my friend. Numerical calculations have this awe-inspiring power, you see. From back in those ancient civilizations to embedding themselves into modern society - it's a testament to our relentless pursuit of knowledge and understanding. It's beautiful, don't you think?

As you dive into your own journey of mastering numerical calculations, my friend, take a moment to appreciate the significance of the past. Look back, learn the lessons, and don't forget the boundless possibilities of the future. With Test Treasure Publication as your trusty guide, we'll give you the tools, insights, and techniques you need to navigate this captivating discipline. Together, my friend, let's venture forth and unlock the hidden treasures that lie within the realm of numerical calculations.

Algebra

Let me take you on a wild ride through the historical timeline of algebra, a real rollercoaster of discoveries and breakthroughs that have totally changed the way we tackle math problems. Buckle up, because this journey begins over two thousand years ago in ancient Babylonia, where these badass scribes were carving mathematical clay tablets like it was nobody's business. These tablets displayed the OG algebraic formulas, the very first recorded instances of them, I might add. These ancient math wizards were all about solving linear and quadratic equations like pros, setting the stage for all the math geeks to come.

Now let's fast forward to Ancient Egypt, where they were getting super fancy with their math. The Rhind Mathematical Papyrus, which dates back to around 1650 BCE, showed off some algebraic moves that would make your head spin. Not only did they rock mathematical problems, but they also showcased this concept called proportional reasoning, which is basically the backbone of algebra. Pretty impressive stuff, right?

The Greeks were no slouches either when it came to algebra. These guys were all about pushing the boundaries and paving the way for future math geniuses. Diophantus, one of the OG Greeks, dropped a masterpiece on us called "Arithmetica" in the third century CE. This bad boy totally revolutionized the game by solving equations with multiple unknowns, creating what we now know as Diophantine equations. At the time, not many people knew about his work, but man, did it lay the foundation for future pioneers in the algebra game.

Now let's talk about the Islamic Golden Age, a time when people's brains were on fire with all things math. Al-Khwarizmi, AKA the "Father of Algebra," was the superstar of this era. This guy championed the advancement of algebraic principles and was dropping knowledge bombs left and right. His treatise, "Al-Kitāb al-Mukhtaṣar fī Ḥisāb al-Jabr wa'l-Muqābala" (can we just take a second to acknowledge how awesome that title is?), not only introduced the concept of algebra but also standardized methods for solving equations. Talk about leaving a lasting legacy!

Fast forward to the Renaissance, and two major players step up to bat: François Viète and René Descartes. These guys completely changed the game. Viète rocked our world by introducing algebraic notation, using letters to represent known and unknown quantities. This move transformed algebra and set the stage for the symbolism that defines modern algebra. Descartes, on the other hand, brought algebra and geometry together like they were long-lost buddies. With the help of his buddy Pierre de Fermat, Descartes developed analytic geometry, this amazing tool that intertwined algebra with geometry. It's like they were saying, "Hey, math, meet math! You guys have a lot in common!"

The 18th and 19th centuries are the peak of mathematical genius, my friend. These guys were on fire. Leonhard Euler and Carl Friedrich Gauss were the tag team that took algebra to new heights. Gauss, in particular, was a straight-up beast. He developed the foundational theories of algebraic number theory, abstract algebra, and the theory of equations. Basically, he opened up a whole new world for future math whizzes to explore. He pushed the limits of Euclidean geometry and made algebra look like a piece of cake.

Here we are, in the present day, and algebra is still blowing our minds. There's so much left to discover and so many wicked concepts and applications just waiting to be unraveled. Here at Test Treasure Publication, we're on a mission to unlock the mysteries of algebra and make it way less intimidating. We're all about demystifying the complexities and giving students the tools to conquer the mathematical universe. So come join us as we dive deeper into the realm of algebra, where equations become irresistible puzzles begging to be solved and variables dance to the rhythm of our mighty intellect.

Probability and Statistics

Step 1: Laying the Foundation

Alright, folks, let's kick off this journey by laying down a solid foundation in the oh-so-important principles of probability. We're about to dive headfirst into the exciting world of chance, where we'll learn how to assign probabilities to different events, understand what it means for something to be independent, and differentiate between discrete and continuous probability distributions. Trust me, once we master the art of calculating probabilities using fancy techniques like combinatorial ones, permutations, and combinations, you'll feel like a statistical superstar ready to tackle more complex problems with confidence.

Step 2: Statistical Inference

Now that we've got probability under our belts, it's time to level up and venture into the world of statistical inference. Get ready to unlock the power of data analysis as we explore some fascinating stuff like sampling, parameter estimation, and hypothesis testing. With these inferential statistics in our back pocket, we'll have the ability to draw meaningful conclusions about whole populations based on limited sample data. We'll even dive into confidence intervals and p-values, revealing the secrets to making informed decisions when things get uncertain.

Step 3: Probability Distributions

As our wild journey continues, we'll come face to face with a whole gang of probability distributions that shape the very fabric of statistical analysis. We've got the fancy normal distribution, the ever-present binomial distribution, and the speedy exponential distribution, each with their own unique story to tell. Once we master these bad boys, we'll have the skills to model and analyze real-world phenomena, extracting meaningful insights from raw data like a boss. And get ready for the Central Limit Theorem to blow your mind, turning a bunch of random variables into a symphony of predictability and patterns.

Step 4: Regression Analysis

In this mind-blowing phase of our journey, we're going to crack the code of regression analysis. We'll learn all about how to model relationships between variables, uncover those hidden patterns, and make predictions with the utmost confidence. We'll start off with the basics of simple linear regression and work our way up to the impressive multiple regression. By the time we're done, you'll have the power to make informed decisions, spot trends from a mile away, and maybe even predict the future (well, sort of).

Step 5: Experimental Design

Hold on tight, folks, because we're now diving into the enchanting realm of experimental design. This is where we learn how to navigate the tricky interplay between dependent and independent variables, control those pesky confounding factors, and extract meaningful conclusions from what seems like a chaotic sea of data. Whether we're dealing with a randomized controlled trial or an observational study, we're giving you the tools to design experiments that yield legit results and pave the way for groundbreaking discoveries. Get ready to become a data detective!

Step 6: Real-World Applications

Now that we're entering the final stretch of our journey, it's time to see how all this probability and statistics magic applies to the real world. We're talking about how these powerful tools impact fields like finance, epidemiology, marketing—you name it. From analyzing risks to ensuring quality control, from making predictive models to decision-making, probability and statistics are everywhere. We're bringing in some captivating case studies to show you the real impact statistical analysis has on society, and trust me, you'll be inspired to use the power of data to shape a better future.

Step 7: Mastery and Beyond

Woohoo! You've made it, my friend. You've conquered the intricate paths of probability and statistics and emerged as a true analysis and inference master. But hold on, this is not the end of the road. At Test Treasure Publication, we believe in continuous growth and evolution. We've got comprehensive resources and ongoing support that'll help you deepen your knowledge, explore advanced topics, and refine your skills to become a statistical virtuoso. So buckle up because there's always more to learn and discover.

Join us on this life-changing expedition through the captivating realm of probability and statistics. Together, we'll unlock the secrets hidden in data, light up the path to extraordinary success, and inspire you to embrace the art of analysis. This journey is just the beginning of a future filled with endless opportunities, where you'll make a profound impact on the world. Welcome to Test Treasure Publication, where the extraordinary becomes the norm, and the adventure never ends.

Geometry

Welcome to the world of Geometry! In this first chapter, we're diving deep into the very foundations of this mind-bending geometric realm. Grab a pen, trace those lines with precision, and get ready to unlock the secrets hidden within points, lines, and planes. It's like unravelling a carefully woven tapestry of intersecting and parallel lines, discovering the hidden symmetries that lie beneath the surface.

But that's just the beginning. Let me be your guide on this enchanting journey through the captivating world of triangles and polygons. We'll explore right triangles that seem to fit perfectly, equilateral ones that radiate balance, and quadrilaterals that somehow contain both order and chaos. And let's not forget about hexagons - those unique creatures with their six sides. Together, we'll unravel the powerful properties that these shapes possess, and trust me, they'll leave you awe-inspired.

Now, hold on tight, because things are about to get even more mesmerizing. We're about to enter the enchanting realm of circles. Picture this: arcs intersecting, tangents dancing gracefully - oh, the drama! And let me tell you, there's more to circles than meets the eye. We'll reveal the secrets behind chords and secants, and you'll be amazed by the radiant beauty of inscribed angles. Trust me, these circles are like their own magical symphony, harmonizing effortlessly with lines, triangles, and other shapes.

But we're not done yet! Hang in there, because our adventure in Geometry is about to take a three-dimensional twist. Get ready to explore the elegance of spheres that seem to envelop everything in smooth grace. We'll admire the edges of pyramids, pointing skyward with their sharp precision. And let's not forget about the prisms - their facets shimmering like diamonds in the sunlight. As we meticulously describe these spatial wonders, you'll start to see the world through a whole new lens.

Now, here's the best part. We're not just here to tell you about these mind-boggling concepts - we want you to experience them for yourself. Test Treasure Publication goes above and beyond by offering a trove of practice problems and interactive exercises. These challenges will put your newfound knowledge to the test, sharpening your geometric prowess and solidifying your understanding. You'll be well-prepared to conquer any geometry-based exam that comes your way!

With Test Treasure as your trusty companion, you'll witness the transformation of Geometry from a daunting labyrinth into a thrilling adventure. We believe that personalized learning, insightful explanations, and a community-driven approach can unlock your full potential. Together, we'll shine in the world of shapes and numbers, reaching extraordinary heights of success.

So, come along and join us at Test Treasure Publication. We're here to illuminate the path to greatness, to invite you on a journey that transcends ordinary learning. Let us be your compass through this enchanting landscape of Geometry, guiding you toward the pinnacle of geometric understanding and academic achievement. The possibilities are endless, my friend. Let's make this journey one for the books!

Trigonometry

Hey there!

So, you know how trigonometry can sometimes feel like this big, mysterious thing? Well, we get it. We've been there too. But here at Test Treasure Publication, we've made it our mission to uncover the secrets of trigonometry and make it accessible and engaging for you.

Angles, my friend, are the building blocks of trigonometry. Understanding how angles work, how they're measured, and how they relate to each other is key to solving all those trigonometric problems. Our study guides go deep into this topic, shedding light on different types of angles, their properties, and why they matter in all those tricky trig calculations.

And let's not forget about the unit circle. This tool is like a secret weapon that connects angles to points on a circle. By understanding the unit circle, you'll gain a profound understanding of trigonometric functions like cosine, sine, and tangent. These functions are the backbone of solving trigonometric equations. Our study materials not only explain them in detail, but also show you how they work in real-life situations. Because let's face it, trigonometry isn't just about numbers and formulas – it's about the world around us.

Triangles, my friend, are also a big part of trigonometry. By understanding the relationships between a triangle's sides and angles, you'll be able to solve all kinds of trig problems. Our study guides break down the different types of triangles and their properties, giving you all the tools you need to tackle problems involving congruence, similarity, and proportions. It's all about building that strong foundation for success.

Here at Test Treasure Publication, we don't just want you to memorize formulas. No way! We want you to truly understand trigonometry and be able to apply your knowledge creatively and confidently. Our study materials are designed to help you do just that. We want you to see the beauty and relevance of trigonometry in the world around us. It's more than just a subject – it's a journey of discovery and inspiration.

So come join us on this journey through the captivating realm of trigonometry. Let us guide you towards success, where this once-mysterious subject becomes your source of inspiration. With our study materials by your side, you'll conquer the complexities of trigonometry like a pro. Are you ready to unlock a world of possibilities and achieve academic excellence? Let's do this!

SECTION 4: THE BIOLOGY

Cellular and Molecular Biology

Welcome, my friends, to the vast and awe-inspiring world of Cellular and Molecular Biology. Here, we are about to embark on a journey that will forever change the way we view life itself. In this realm, we discover two intertwined worlds that shape the very fabric of existence: the cellular level and the molecular level.

Let's start at the cellular level, where we step into a universe of breathtaking beauty and intricate machinery. Within every tiny cell, the building blocks of life, lies a world of wonder. It is a place where organelles, membranes, and cytoplasmic activities harmonize to create the magic of life. Take a moment to picture it - a powerhouse within the cell known as the mitochondria, fueled by the energy of life itself, producing the precious ATP molecules that bring vitality to all the biological processes occurring within. It's like a bustling city, with genetic information swirling within the nucleus, as DNA is transformed into RNA and proteins, the architects of life's blueprint. And don't forget the ribosomes in the cytoplasm, working tirelessly to synthesize proteins, the messengers that carry out the cell's wishes. It's a symphony of complexity and coordination, all working together to sustain the delicate harmony of life.

Now let's journey into the molecular level, where we witness the enchanting dance of atoms and their electrifying transformation into molecules. Here, chemical reactions unfold like an elegant ballet, guided by enzymes, the heroes that make life possible. Our attention is captured by the magnificent structure of DNA, the mastermind behind the genetic code that allows for inheritance and diversity. And as we delve deeper into the world of molecular genetics, we unlock the language of genes, deciphering the code that determines the traits that make each organism one-of-a-kind. Ah, and the wonder of protein synthesis! Amino acids coming together to form complex chains that fold and twist, giving rise to the intricate three-dimensional structures that define the functions of life.

As we navigate the complexities of Cellular and Molecular Biology, we can't help but be in awe of the unity that stretches across scales. From the minute world of cells to the molecular intricacies that shape life's grandeur, there is a harmony and interconnectedness that underlies the diversity of living organisms. The processes, the structures, the interactions - they all combine to form a symphony that sustains the beauty and complexity of life.

Here at Test Treasure Publication, we are here to be your guides in the fascinating world of Cellular and Molecular Biology. Our study materials have been lovingly crafted to not only impart knowledge but also to nurture a deep understanding of the wonders within this realm. From our uniquely designed flashcards to our comprehensive study guides and online resources, we are here to accompany you on this thrilling adventure into the labyrinth of cellular processes, molecular structures, and genetic mechanisms. We believe that by shedding light on the intricate world of Cellular and Molecular Biology, we ignite a lifelong passion for learning and inspire the next generation of innovators and researchers.

So, my friends, are you ready to embark on this captivating journey into the realms of Cellular and Molecular Biology? A journey where the microscopic world holds the keys to unlocking the magnificence of life itself? Let us join hands as we unravel the mysteries, ignite our curiosity, and celebrate the wonders that lie within this captivating realm. Together, let us embark on this adventure of a lifetime.

Diversity of Life

1: The Tree of Life

Come with me, my friends, as we immerse ourselves in an enchanting journey through the dazzling web of life on our extraordinary planet. From the tiniest creatures that escape our vision to the awe-inspiring grandeur of majestic beings, we will explore the magnificent diversity that makes our world so breathtaking. Join me, won't you, on this voyage of discovery as we unravel the mysteries of life's origin and uncover the countless species that call every corner of our Earth their home.

2: Exploring Microscopic Worlds

Now, my fellow adventurers, prepare to venture into the hidden realms of the minuscule. In this chapter, we will peer through the lens of a microscope and find ourselves immersed in a world of spellbinding diversity. From the resilient bacteria thriving in the harshest environments to the elusive beauty of viruses, we will uncover the hidden complexity that thrives within these microscopic organisms. Together, my friends, we will unravel the significance of these invisible heroes in our world - their essential roles in ecosystems and their profound impact on human well-being.

3: Unveiling the Secrets of the Plant Kingdom

Step with me, my companions, into a realm bursting with life and colors. As we enter the vibrant world of plants, prepare to be swept away by a kaleidoscope of hues, textures, and fragrances. In this chapter, we will explore the wealth of plant species that grace our Earth - from towering trees in the lush rainforests, to delicate wildflowers swaying in meadows, and resilient succulents that thrive in unforgiving deserts. Brace yourselves, my friends, as we uncover the miracles of photosynthesis, delve into the astounding adaptations that plants have developed, and comprehend the vital role they play in sustaining life on our precious planet.

4: The Animal Kingdom: From Tiny Invertebrates to Majestic Mammals

Hold your breath, my dear companions, as we prepare to encounter the extraordinary realm of animals. From the microscopic intricacies of sponges and jellyfish to the breathtaking splendor of elephants and whales, prepare to have your senses ignited. Through captivating tales and vivid descriptions, we will embark on a journey through the diverse body structures, behaviors, and habitats of these incredible creatures. Prepare yourselves for an escapade that will take us from the darkest depths of the oceans to the towering peaks of mountains, as we uncover the vastness and diversity of the animal kingdom.

5: Understanding Human Diversity

In this momentous final chapter, let us turn our gaze inward and delve into the remarkable diversity within our own species, the Homo sapiens. As sentient beings, we possess a unique power to mold our own destinies, forging diverse cultures, traditions, and belief systems. Together, my dear friends, let us explore the captivating factors that contribute to human diversity - from the intricate dance between genetics and environment to the profound influence of culture. By celebrating and embracing our differences, we foster understanding, compassion, and a world that cherishes unity in the face of diversity.

As we journey through the pages of this comprehensive exploration, let us remember that we have merely scratched the surface of nature's magnificent tapestry. My dear friends, I implore you to keep an open mind, to marvel at the wonders that life has to offer, and to treasure the immense diversity that envelops us. So, come, let us embark together on this transcendental voyage, inspired by the breathtaking beauty and interconnectedness of the world we call home.

Structure and Functions of Systems

Come on, let's take a trip through time and unravel the mind-blowing tale of our magnificent bodies. It all goes back to those ancient civilizations, ya know? Picture this: ancient Egypt, where they thought the heart was the place where all that thinking and feeling happened. Then in ancient India, those Ayurvedic texts were all about how everything in our bodies is connected and intertwined. They were laying down the foundations of what we now know about human anatomy and how our bodies work.

But let's fast forward a bit to the Renaissance era. This is when things really start getting exciting. People like Leonardo da Vinci were totally obsessed with figuring out how our bodies ticked. I mean, this dude was drawing anatomical masterpieces left and right, pushing the boundaries of what we knew about ourselves. He and other visionaries were the real OG scientists, paving the way for the scientific exploration that was about to go down.

Then, in the 17th century, boom! Enter the microscope. Suddenly, we could see a whole microscopic world that our eyes had never laid eyes on before. Scientists like Robert Hooke and Antonie van Leeuwenhoek blew our minds with their discoveries about the intricate inner workings of our cells. These guys were the ones who showed us how our cells work together and make up the foundation of life itself.

And the discoveries just kept coming, one after another, like a never-ending wave. The 19th century brought us the concept of homeostasis, all thanks to this dude named Claude Bernard. He showed us that our bodies have this amazing ability to maintain balance no matter what kind of crazy stuff is going on around us. It's like a delicate dance of stability in the midst of a constantly changing environment.

As time went on, technology started getting fancier. X-rays, electrocardiograms, and all sorts of other cool gadgets allowed us to see what was really going on inside our bodies. We could get a glimpse of the intricate architecture that makes up our organs and tissues, and we started to understand what makes everything function the way it does.

So here we are, in the present day, standing on the shoulders of these brilliant giants who came before us. We have so much knowledge and so many tools at our disposal to explore our bodies with such unbelievable precision. It's like we're detectives, diving into the cardiovascular system, unraveling the mysteries of those mighty vessels and the pumping powerhouse that is our heart. We're digging deep into the respiratory system, witnessing the delicate exchange of oxygen and carbon dioxide that keeps us alive and kickin'. We're in awe of the digestive system, watching as food gets broken down and transformed into the building blocks of life that keep us going strong.

And it doesn't stop there, my friends. The nervous system blows us away with its complex network of neurons, zapping messages at lightning speed, controlling every move, sensation, and thought. And let's not forget about those muscles. They're like superheroes, propelling our bodies through space with their incredible strength and agility.

But here's the thing, guys. As we explore all these systems, we start to realize that they're not just separate little teams doing their own thing. Oh no, they're like this harmonious orchestra, all working together and depending on each other. It's like this crazy intricate dance of signals, chemicals, and energy, all coming together to keep us alive and kicking.

So, here we are, ready to take you on this wild adventure through the human body. We want you to be amazed by the complexity. We want you to be blown away by the beauty that lies within all of us. So grab onto your seats, my friends, because we're about to unlock the secrets of life itself. Get ready to journey with us, where knowledge becomes wisdom, and understanding transforms mere curiosity into sheer awe. Together, let's explore the wonders of the human body and dive into the true treasure that lies within.

Genetics

Here at Test Treasure Publication, we totally get how important genetics is when it comes to rocking the scientific game. Like seriously, this branch of biology is the key to understanding how we inherit traits, how evolution works, and what makes life tick. And that's why we've worked hard to put together a super-duper study guide that will give students the power to conquer the wild world of genetics with confidence and excitement!

So in our awesome study guide, we take a deep dive into the inner workings of cells and how they hook us up with our genes. We follow the twists and turns of DNA, figuring out its crazy double helix structure and decoding the secrets that shape who we are and where we come from. We've got tons of cool illustrations and explanations that make genetics way more fun and easy to understand, so students can really see how amazing this stuff is.

But hey, genetics isn't just about knowing the basics. It's all about how genes, our environment, and evolution come together and do their thing. That's why we're all about exploring the ins and outs of gene regulation. We want students to get a grip on how genes can get switched on or off, and how that leads to all the different traits that make us unique. And we don't stop there – we also shine a light on genetic disorders and what happens when mutations and abnormalities mess with our genes. We dive deep into case studies so students can really see how genetics affects our health and society as a whole. It's like, genetics is everywhere, man!

But we ain't done yet, my friend. At Test Treasure Publication, we know that true learning happens when you put what you know into action. That's why our study guide isn't just about reading - we've got loads of interactive exercises and discussion questions that make students really think and apply what they've learned. We want students to be awesome critical thinkers, you know? And to truly get genetics inside and out.

As I sit here and think about how dang important genetics is in the big ol' world of science, I'm blown away by its crazy potential. From unlocking the secrets of inheritance to finding sick new ways to treat diseases, genetics is a game-changer. And we're totally stoked to be on this journey with our students, sparking a love for genetics that goes way beyond just school stuff.

So come on, let's go on this mind-blowing adventure into the world of genetics together. We're gonna untangle the mysteries of life, find out what makes us who we are, and have a blast exploring the incredible ways genes can mix and match. Test Treasure Publication is gonna be your guide on this rad quest, where the ordinary becomes extraordinary, and where we light the way to success in the totally mind-blowing realm of genetics. Let's do this!

Evolution, Ecology, and Behavior

Let's dive deep into the captivating world of evolution. It's not just some scientific concept - it's a symphony of life that's been playing for billions of years. With our study materials, we'll peel back the layers of this ancient melody and reveal the intricacies that have shaped the diversity we see today.

We'll take you back to the very beginning - the dawn of life itself. We'll explore the origins of the first organisms and the forces that transformed them. From simple microorganisms to the mind-blowing complexity of modern species, we'll unravel the threads of evolutionary history that connect us all.

Next stop: the web of ecology. Think of it like being a skilled detective. We'll guide you through the intricacies of the ecological web and unveil its mysteries one thread at a time. Our study guides will teach you about the delicate balance of ecosystems, the dance between organisms and their surroundings, and how life adapts and thrives in diverse environments. We'll take you on a virtual journey to witness the wonders of our planet's interconnectedness, from towering forests to the bottom of the ocean.

Now let's decode behavioral patterns. Behaviors are like windows into living beings. They give us a glimpse into their inner workings. In this section, we'll delve into the fascinating realm of animal behavior, uncovering the motives and strategies that drive their actions. Our comprehensive flashcards and study materials will introduce you to the theories and concepts that form the foundation of behavioral biology. We'll explore the intricacies of communication, social structures, mating rituals, and survival strategies. Each action tells a story waiting to be deciphered - prepare to be captivated!

Finally, we'll connect the threads that make up the grand tapestry of life. Evolution, ecology, and behavior are all intertwined, forming a holistic understanding of the living world. With our guidance, you'll gain a comprehensive understanding of how evolution shapes behavior and ecological interactions. You'll learn to recognize patterns and processes that have driven the adaptation and survival of species over time. Armed with this knowledge, you'll be better equipped to navigate the natural world and appreciate the beauty and complexity of life in all its forms.

Join us on this journey of discovery and enlightenment. Let's unravel the mysteries of the natural world and uncover the secrets that have shaped the living beings we share this planet with. Evolution, ecology, and behavior - where the past meets the present, where the threads of life seamlessly intertwine. Get ready for an adventure!

Section 5: The General Chemistry

States of Matter

Welcome to this chapter, my friend. Get ready for an incredible journey into the mysterious world of states of matter. We're about to uncover the secrets behind how different substances behave and the physical properties that make them unique. From the comforting warmth of a steaming cup of tea to the mesmerizing dance of molecules during a thunderstorm, we'll explore the wonders all around us.

Let's start with the Solid State - a realm that may seem motionless, but holds incredible strength and stability within it. Picture a grand fortress standing strong, protecting us from the chaos outside. We'll dive into the crystalline lattices that make up solids, discovering what gives them their rigid structure and the forces that hold them together. Get ready to witness the mind-blowing phenomenon of polymorphism, where a substance can exist in multiple solid forms, each with its own special properties.

Now, let's move on to Liquids - where freedom takes the center stage. Imagine a symphony in motion, with molecules gracefully dancing, unrestricted by the solid's rigidity. In this chapter, we'll unravel the dynamics of intermolecular attractions within liquids, unlocking their unique properties like viscosity and surface tension. And get this - we'll explore the magic of capillary action, where liquids defy gravity, and the enchanting world of phase diagrams, where temperature and pressure define which state of matter we're in.

The adventure doesn't stop there. We still have Gases to conquer. Brace yourself for the wild and chaotic dance of molecules, colliding and bouncing off one another, filled with boundless energy. In this chapter, we'll unlock the fundamental principles behind how gases behave. The ideal gas law will be our guide as we examine how temperature, pressure, and volume interact to shape gas behavior. And prepare to be amazed by the wonders of diffusion, where gases effortlessly mix and spread, and the captivating dance of effusion, where they escape through minuscule openings, almost invisible to the naked eye.

Get ready for the grand finale - Phase Transitions. It's a breathtaking spectacle where matter transforms from one state to another. Imagine a delicate snowflake melting into a shimmering droplet or the mesmerizing dance of water vapor condensing into a cloudy sky. In this final chapter, we'll witness the incredible journeys that matter takes during these transitions. From melting and freezing to evaporation and condensation, we'll delve deep into the secrets that govern these transformations.

As we come to the end of this chapter, take a moment to reflect on all the knowledge and wonders we've discovered. This journey through the states of matter has given us a glimpse into the extraordinary world that lies beneath the surface of our daily lives. And remember, my friend, studying matter isn't just about reaching an end goal; it's an opportunity to appreciate the beauty and complexity of the universe we inhabit. So, embrace this newfound knowledge and let it guide you not only in your academic pursuits but also in your pursuit of an extraordinary life.

As we bid adieu to the exploration of states of matter, I invite you to take what you've learned and weave it into the fabric of your understanding. Let this knowledge shape your future endeavors and guide you towards extraordinary success. Until we meet again, remember that at Test Treasure Publication, our mission is to light up the path to success and embark on a journey of learning that goes beyond the ordinary.

Solutions

Alright, here's what you need to do to ace your exams.

Step 1: Assess and Analyze. Take a moment to figure out where you stand. Our online assessment tools and diagnostic tests give you a clear picture of what you're good at and what needs work. We dig deep into your strengths and weaknesses, so you know exactly where to focus your efforts.

Step 2: Personalized Study Plan. Armed with the results from the assessment, we create a study plan that's tailor-made just for you. Think of it as a roadmap to success. Our study guides break down complex topics into bite-sized pieces, making it easier for you to understand and learn. Trust us, every study session will be worth your while.

Step 3: Interactive Learning. Forget about boring lectures and textbooks. We believe in making learning fun and engaging. Our flashcards and online study materials turn memorization into an exciting adventure. We've got interactive quizzes, visual aids, and multimedia resources to make sure you enjoy the journey while mastering the material.

Step 4: Practice, Practice, Practice. You know the saying, right? Practice makes perfect. That's why we've compiled a comprehensive collection of practice tests that will push your limits, challenge your thinking, and sharpen your skills. These practice questions are designed to mimic the real deal, so you'll feel confident and comfortable on exam day.

Step 5: Continuous Feedback and Improvement. We're all about growth and progress. Our study materials come with built-in feedback systems that give you real-time insights into your performance. Our algorithms analyze your strengths and weaknesses, so you'll know exactly where to focus your efforts. We'll also give you tailored recommendations for improvement because we want to see you succeed.

Step 6: Community Support. No one should go through this journey alone. That's why we've created a supportive community for all our students. Join our online forums and discussion boards to connect with like-minded peers, get advice from experienced mentors, and share your wins and struggles. Together, we'll lift each other up and achieve greatness.

Step 7: Last-Minute Preparation. When the exam day is creeping closer, we've got your back. We offer last-minute resources to help you review and polish your knowledge and skills. Our review guides and cheat sheets are quick refreshers that give you just what you need to tackle any challenge that comes your way.

Step 8: Conquer the Exam. Now it's time to show off all your hard work. With our comprehensive study materials, personalized approach, and community support, you're ready to conquer any exam that comes your way. Walk into that exam room with confidence and grace, knowing that you've got what it takes to succeed.

At Test Treasure Publication, we're all about helping you reach your goals. Our step-by-step guide is just one part of our commitment to empowering you in your academic journey. Let's embark on this extraordinary adventure together and uncover the endless possibilities that lie within you.

Kinetics and Equilibrium

Come step into this fantastical world with me, where time dances and swirls, controlling the speed at which amazing reactions happen. Imagine a place where catalysts possess the power to wield magic, speeding up the transformation of reactants into products with the most incredible efficiency. Get ready to peel back these layers of complexity, my friend, and develop a deep understanding of how factors like reactant concentration and collision temperature influence reaction rates.

But hold on tight, because just when you thought the enchantment couldn't get any greater, equilibrium comes calling. It's like nature walking a tightrope, delicately balancing the forward and reverse reactions so they occur at the same rate. Picture this equilibrium taking shape amidst the chaos of chemical reactions, where the reactants strive for control while the products fight to claim their rightful place.

Now, prepare yourself for a deep dive into the laws that rule this equilibrium realm. We'll unravel the wisdom of Le Chatelier, a genius who sheds light on systems in equilibrium. You'll see how a change in pressure, temperature, or concentration can tip the balance, shifting reactions to favor either the forward or the reverse direction.

But remember, my friend, this adventure isn't one you have to face alone. As we journey through this captivating world, we'll tap into the power of collaboration and shared knowledge. At Test Treasure Publication, we believe in creating a vibrant community of learners, where insights are freely shared, questions are eagerly answered, and those moments of epiphany are celebrated like fireworks in the night sky. Together, we will plunge into the depths of kinetics and equilibrium, buoyed by the support of our fellow explorers.

Get ready to have your socks knocked off, because in this world of kinetics and equilibrium, magic is in the air. With the guidance of Test Treasure Publication, you'll transcend the dry pages of a textbook and discover the breathtaking beauty that lies within the realm of chemical reactions. So, dear reader, buckle up and embrace this extraordinary journey, where ordinary learning is left at the dock, and an extraordinary understanding takes flight. The secrets of kinetics and equilibrium await your eager mind. Let's set sail, my friend, and embark on this awe-inspiring voyage together.

Atomic and Molecular Structure

Let's start by diving into the fascinating world of atoms. I mean, seriously, these tiny little things are the building blocks of everything around us! They make up the air we breathe, the ground we walk on, and even the food we eat. It's mind-boggling to think about.

Atoms are like these super exclusive clubs where only a few subatomic particles are allowed in. We've got protons, which are all about positivity, neutrons, who are just kind of chill, and electrons, the negative charge bearers. Together, they form the nucleus of the atom, like the VIP section, while the electrons twirl around it like party-goers on a dance floor.

Alright, buckle up, because we're about to meet molecules. Picture this: atoms decide to hold hands and form these cool little groups called molecules. It's like the ultimate chemistry bonding session. They can either go for the full-on TV drama type of bonding, called ionic bonding, or keep it casual with covalent bonding.

Ionic bonding is like that intense relationship where one atom just can't let go of its electrons. It's a total transfer of power, creating these charged species called ions. On the other hand, covalent bonding is like being best friends who share everything. The atoms share their electrons, creating stable molecular compounds, no fights or drama involved.

Now, let's venture into the world of electron configuration. Picture the nucleus of an atom as a fancy nightclub surrounded by different levels or orbitals occupied by electrons. These electrons follow some serious rules dictated by quantum mechanics. These rules determine the atom's stability and behavior, like when to go for a dance and when to just chill by the bar.

Atoms and molecules are more than just their makeup. They have their own unique personalities, like electronegativity, atomic radius, and ionization energy. These traits have a huge impact on the way they react and interact with other atoms and molecules. It's like a chemistry version of a personality test.

Oh, and we can't forget about the epic phenomenon of hybridization. It's like atoms getting a total makeover. Atomic orbitals decide to mix and match, creating new orbitals that then bond with other atoms. It's like a chemistry version of Project Runway, where the final outcome is a perfectly stable compound with killer style and geometry.

Let's not leave out the rockstar of the show - quantum mechanics. This is where things get real trippy. Quantum mechanics is like the backstage pass to the show. It allows us to understand the crazy behavior of electrons and how they distribute themselves in atoms and molecules. It's like peering behind the curtain and watching the magic happen.

So, time to prepare for the adventure of a lifetime. We're about to unravel the secrets of the microscopic world and witness things that will leave you in awe. Get ready to appreciate and understand the complexities of our universe, because it's about to get mind-blowing. Together, we'll conquer the DAT and beyond, unlocking the wisdom that lies within the incredible world of atomic and molecular structure. Let's do this!

SECTION 6: THE ORGANIC CHEMISTRY

Chemical

and Physical Properties of Molecules

Alright, my friend, let's dive into the fascinating world of chemical properties. We're about to unravel the mysteries behind how substances react with each other. It's like watching atoms and molecules tango, forming and breaking bonds right before our eyes. Get ready to have your mind blown.

Now, hold on tight because things are about to get interesting. We're going to talk about electronegativity and oxidation states. These concepts are like our trusty compasses, helping us predict how elements and compounds behave. It's wild how electronegativity affects the way bonds form, and it's even crazier how oxidation and reduction reactions are complete opposites.

But wait, there's more! We haven't even touched on the physical properties of molecules. We're going to explore the characteristics we can observe and measure without messing with the chemical composition. Stuff like boiling points, melting points, vapor pressure, and solubility. You won't believe the forces that control these mind-boggling phenomena.

Speaking of forces, get ready to dive into the underworld of intermolecular forces. We're going to uncover the secrets behind hydrogen bonding, dipole-dipole interactions, and London dispersion forces. These sneaky forces determine why different substances behave the way they do. It's like a secret language that only molecules understand.

Now, hold your breath because we're entering the captivating world of spectroscopy. We're going to analyze how molecules interact with different types of electromagnetic radiation. From ultraviolet-visible spectroscopy to infrared spectroscopy, we'll decode the spectral fingerprints of substances. It's like solving a thrilling mystery and uncovering the true identity of molecules.

But hey, we're not just going to sit back and read. We're going to get our hands dirty with experiments and simulations. We'll witness incredible transformations, observe physical changes, and be amazed by the power of understanding these properties. It's time to put our knowledge to the test and see the wonders we can unlock.

As our journey comes to an end, we realize that this isn't just limited to the classroom. Our understanding of these chemical and physical properties opens up a whole new world of possibilities. From groundbreaking pharmaceutical research to revolutionary materials science to saving the environment, we have the power to make a real impact with our newfound knowledge.

So, my dear reader, welcome to this captivating chapter of our book. Together, we're embarking on an eye-opening expedition through the complex tapestry of chemical and physical properties of molecules. By the time we reach the final page, you'll have a deep understanding and appreciation for the incredible world that lies right at the heart of all matter. So, let's set off on this thrilling adventure and unlock the secrets that await us.

Nomenclature

Alright, folks, let's dive right into the mesmerizing realm of nomenclature. This fancy word basically means the science of naming stuff. And trust me, it's way cooler than it sounds. It's like this secret language, a key that unlocks the door to understanding all sorts of disciplines. As wannabe scholars, we gotta embrace this language with open arms, 'cause it's through nomenclature that we really connect with our chosen field of study.

Here at Test Treasure Publication, we totally get how important nomenclature is for academic success. We believe that if you can master the art of naming things, you've pretty much got the power to breeze through the endless sea of knowledge. With nomenclature, you get to explore Latin and Greek roots that lay the foundation of scientific terms, and even get into the fancy systems used to classify living things. It's like a bridge connecting all the fancy ideas with real-world understanding.

So, buckle up, 'cause in this chapter we're going on a mind-blowing journey through the world of nomenclature. We'll explore its origins, its purpose, and how it shapes our academic adventures. This ain't just about acquiring knowledge, my friends, it's about mastering a skill that'll guide our intellectual journey.

Moving on to Step 1: Navigating the Nomenclature of Science

Science, with all its branches and sub-disciplines, can be a bit overwhelming, especially for beginners. But fear not, my friends! We're here to guide you through the fascinating world of scientific nomenclature and give you the tools to crack its secret code.

Each branch of science has its own special nomenclature. From elements in chemistry to the different types of organisms in biology, there's a whole system of naming stuff. And guess what? Scientists use this precise language to communicate with each other, not just today but throughout history. By mastering the rules and conventions of scientific nomenclature, you become part of a conversation that's been going on for centuries. Talk about leaving your mark on the tapestry of knowledge!

In this chapter, we're gonna uncover the secrets of scientific nomenclature. We'll break down all its complicated bits and make sure you get it all. We'll explore how different things are classified, explain the rules of fancy terms like binomial nomenclature, and even show you how scientific names are created. We'll make it all vivid, engaging, and interactive, so you can navigate through the crazy world of scientific language like a boss.

On to Step 2: Navigating the Nomenclature of Medicine

Alright, let's talk medicine! This field is all about saving lives and making a difference, and guess what? Its nomenclature is just as crucial as the treatments. In this step, we're gonna take a mind-blowing journey through the world of medical nomenclature.

In medicine, nomenclature has a twofold purpose. It helps medical professionals communicate with each other using a language that everyone understands. And it also gives patients and the community a sense of trust and assurance. By speaking this language fluently, you become a beacon of healing and comfort.

So, in this chapter, we're diving deep into the intricacies of medical nomenclature. We'll explore all the fancy anatomical terms, those medical abbreviations that make you go, "What the heck?!" and even dive into diagnostic codes. But fear not, we'll make it fun and interactive with exercises and real-life case studies. You'll be able to unravel the complexity of this language and communicate effectively in the world of medicine.

And finally, Step 3: Navigating the Nomenclature of Mathematics

Now it's time to tackle the mysterious world of mathematics. Some call it the language of the universe, others call it the land of numbers. Either way, its nomenclature is like a special code that gives us unparalleled precision and logical reasoning. In this last step, we're gonna immerse ourselves in the amazing world of mathematical nomenclature and learn to understand the language of numbers.

Within the realm of mathematics, nomenclature plays a crucial role in expressing abstract concepts in a precise way. It's through this language that mathematicians share their theories, discoveries, and proofs. By mastering the nomenclature of mathematics, you'll join the ranks of brilliant minds who explore the mysteries of the universe with analytical and creative thinking.

In this chapter, we're gonna embark on an exhilarating adventure into mathematical nomenclature. We'll uncover the hidden meanings behind all those symbols and formulas that initially make your head spin. We'll cover everything from algebra to geometry, calculus, and beyond. And don't worry, we'll make it super engaging with examples, step-by-step explanations, and even some mind-bending puzzles. Get ready to appreciate the elegance and power of mathematical nomenclature like never before!

So, my friends, keep exploring the pages of Test Treasure Publication's DAT Prep Book. Together, we'll light up the path to extraordinary success, turning the seemingly ordinary into an adventure of learning and discovery. Join us as we unlock the secrets, master the art, and become the torchbearers of knowledge in the academic world.

Functional Group Chemistry

1. Introduction to Functional Groups:

Imagine yourself stepping into the captivating world of functional groups. These awesome clusters of atoms hold the key to the reactivity and properties of organic compounds. From the bold aromas of aldehydes that waft through the air, to the elegant double bonds of alkenes that dance through molecules, each functional group gives a unique identity to a compound. In this chapter, get ready to unravel the secrets of these influential groups, and equip yourself with the tools to understand, analyze, and manipulate their magical organic powers.

2. Alcohols and Ethers:

Raise your glass as we dive into the fascinating realm of alcohols and ethers. Imagine alcohols with their hydroxyl groups, versatile and celebrated in a multitude of ways. Ethanol reigns as the elixir of celebrations, while methanol powers up our engines. And then there are ethers, always adding that touch of mystery to organic structures with their oxygen atom linked to two hydrocarbon groups. Together, we will uncover their captivating properties, decode their names, and explore the intoxicating allure of alcohols and ethers.

3. Aldehydes and Ketones:

Get ready to awaken your olfactory senses and experience the delightful world of aldehydes and ketones. Aldehydes, with their carbonyl group attached to a hydrogen atom, fill the air with the mouthwatering aroma of freshly baked pastries. Ketones, on the other hand, exude elegance, with their carbonyl groups nestled between two hydrocarbon groups. We will journey through their reactivity, learn their naming conventions, and uncover their pivotal role in synthesizing organic compounds. Hold on tight, because the scents and charm of aldehydes and ketones are about to transport you to a whole new dimension.

4. Carboxylic Acids and Esters:

Welcome to the symphony of acidity and sweetness in the realm of carboxylic acids and esters. Carboxylic acids, with their carboxyl groups, give vinegar its sharp scent and contribute to the tangy flavors of fruits. Esters, on the other hand, bless us with the enchanting scent of flowers and the tantalizing allure of perfumes. As we embark on this journey, we will unlock the art of naming these compounds, dive into their unique reactions, and explore the vast possibilities they offer in the world of organic synthesis. Get ready to be captivated by the dance of acidity and sweetness.

5. Amines and Amides:

Step into the realm where nitrogen atoms take center stage, and everything feels fresh and vibrant. Amines, with their nitrogen substituents, infuse a wide array of organic compounds with a refreshing burst of life. Amides, on the other hand, reveal themselves as the resilient backbone of proteins, binding us to the wonders of life itself. Together, we will navigate their classification, unravel their naming conventions, and delve into their fundamental role in biological systems. Join us on this enlightening journey, where nitrogen bonds will bring a new wave of excitement to your understanding of functional groups.

6. Alkenes and Alkynes:

Prepare yourself to take flight as we enter the realm of unsaturated hydrocarbons. Alkenes, with their captivating double bonds, open up a world of endless possibilities for diverse reactions, unleashing the creative potential within us. Alkynes, with their triple bonds, stand tall as the stable and reactive targets that synthetic chemists around the globe pine for. We will uncover the intricacies of their structural features, decode their names, and dive into their transformative power in the realm of organic chemistry. Buckle up for an exhilarating ride through the world of double and triple bonds.

7. Aromatic Compounds:

Finally, we arrive at the grand finale - the mesmerizing world of aromatic compounds. Picture aromatic rings weaving a tapestry of captivating scents and exquisite chemical reactivity. From the alluring fragrance of benzene to the medicinal properties of aspirin, aromatic compounds occupy a central place in the realm of chemistry. Brace yourself as we explore their reactivity, decode their names, and uncover the fascinating historical significance that surrounds this remarkable class of compounds. Get ready to be swept off your feet by the wonders and mysteries of aromatic compounds.

At Test Treasure Publications, we invite you to embark on this exhilarating odyssey through the realm of functional group chemistry. Let our meticulously crafted study materials be your guiding light, illuminating the path to extraordinary success in your DAT exam preparation. Together, we will unravel the intricacies of functional groups, empowering you with the knowledge to conquer any challenge that comes your way. So, join us on this enlightening journey and watch your understanding of functional group chemistry bloom like a budding flower in the vast garden of organic chemistry.

FULL-LENGTH PRACTICE TEST 1

Section 1: The Perceptual Ability

1. Apertures

Question 1: Which shape would result from passing a cube through a circular aperture?
A) Circle
B) Square
C) Rectangle
D) Triangle

Answer: B) Square
Explanation: A cube would create a square shape when passed through a circular aperture as the aperture captures the cross-sectional area of the cube, which is square.

2. View Recognition

Question 2: From the top view, how many faces of a cube can be seen?
A) 1
B) 2

C) 3

D) 4

Answer: A) 1

Explanation: From a top view, only the top face of the cube is visible.

3. Angle Discrimination

Question 3: What is the measure of each interior angle in an equilateral triangle?

A) 45°

B) 60°

C) 90°

D) 120°

Answer: B) 60°

Explanation: In an equilateral triangle, each interior angle is 60°.

4. Paper Folding

Question 4: If you fold a square paper in half, what shape will you get?

A) Triangle

B) Rectangle

C) Pentagon

D) Circle

Answer: B) Rectangle

Explanation: Folding a square paper in half will result in a rectangle.

5. Cube Counting

Question 5: How many cubes are there in a 3x3x3 cube structure?

A) 9

B) 18

C) 27

D) 36

Answer: C) 27

Explanation: A 3x3x3 cube structure contains 27 individual cubes.

6. 3D Form Development

Question 6: Which 3D shape is formed by revolving a rectangle around its longer side?

A) Sphere

B) Cylinder

C) Cone

D) Pyramid

Answer: B) Cylinder

Explanation: Revolving a rectangle around its longer side will create a cylinder.

Section 2: The Reading Comprehension

7. Comprehension Skills

Question 7: What is the main idea of a story called the "thesis"?

A) True

B) False

Answer: B) False

Explanation: The main idea of a story is not called the thesis; it's usually referred to as the "theme" or "central idea."

8. Critical Thinking Skills

Question 8: Which of the following is an example of an assumption?
A) The sun rises in the east.
B) All humans breathe.
C) If it's raining, the ground will be wet.
D) Water boils at 100°C.

Answer: C) If it's raining, the ground will be wet
Explanation: This statement assumes that the ground will be wet if it's raining, without considering other factors like absorption or drainage.

Section 3: The Quantitative Reasoning

9. Numerical Calculations

Question 9: What is the square root of 81?
A) 8
B) 9
C) 10
D) 11

Answer: B) 9
Explanation: The square root of 81 is 9.

10. Algebra

Question 10: Solve for x: $2x + 3 = 11$
A) 2
B) 3

C) 4

D) 5

Answer: C) 4

Explanation: Solving the equation $2x + 3 = 11$ gives $x = 4$.

11. Probability and Statistics

Question 11: What is the probability of rolling a 3 on a standard 6-sided die?

A) 1/2

B) 1/3

C) 1/4

D) 1/6

Answer: D) 1/6

Explanation: There is one 3 on a 6-sided die, so the probability is 1/6.

12. Geometry

Question 12: What is the sum of the interior angles of a triangle?

A) 90°

B) 180°

C) 270°

D) 360°

Answer: B) 180°

Explanation: The sum of the interior angles of a triangle is 180°.

13. Trigonometry

Question 13: What is the sine of 90 degrees?

A) 0

B) 0.5

C) 1

D) 1.5

Answer: C) 1

Explanation: The sine of 90 degrees is 1.

Section 4: The Biology

14. Cellular and Molecular Biology

Question 14: What is the powerhouse of the cell?

A) Nucleus

B) Ribosome

C) Mitochondria

D) Endoplasmic Reticulum

Answer: C) Mitochondria

Explanation: The mitochondria are often referred to as the "powerhouse of the cell" as they produce ATP, the cell's energy currency.

15. Diversity of Life

Question 15: Which of the following is a mammal?

A) Shark

B) Sparrow

C) Human

D) Frog

Answer: C) Human

Explanation: Humans are mammals.

16. Structure and Functions of Systems

Question 16: Which organ is responsible for filtering blood in the human body?
A) Heart
B) Kidney
C) Liver
D) Lungs

Answer: B) Kidney
Explanation: The kidneys are responsible for filtering blood.

17. Genetics

Question 17: What is the dominant trait in Mendel's pea plant experiments?
A) Yellow color
B) Green color
C) Tall height
D) Short height

Answer: A) Yellow color
Explanation: In Mendel's experiments, yellow was the dominant color for pea plants.

18. Evolution, Ecology, and Behavior

Question 18: What term describes the behavior of animals that live in groups for mutual benefit?
A) Hibernation
B) Solitary
C) Symbiosis
D) Social

Answer: D) Social

Explanation: Animals that live in groups for mutual benefit exhibit social behavior.

Section 5: The General Chemistry

19. States of Matter

Question 19: What state of matter has a definite shape and volume?

A) Liquid

B) Solid

C) Gas

D) Plasma

Answer: B) Solid

Explanation: Solids have a definite shape and volume.

20. Solutions

Question 20: What is the solute in a sugar water solution?

A) Water

B) Sugar

C) Neither

D) Both

Answer: B) Sugar

Explanation: In a sugar water solution, sugar is the solute.

21. Kinetics and Equilibrium

Question 21: What factor affects the rate of a chemical reaction?

A) Temperature

B) Color

C) Taste

D) Smell

Answer: A) Temperature

Explanation: Temperature is a factor that can affect the rate of a chemical reaction.

22. Atomic and Molecular Structure

Question 22: What is the atomic number of helium?

A) 1

B) 2

C) 3

D) 4

Answer: B) 2

Explanation: The atomic number of helium is 2.

Section 6: The Organic Chemistry

23. Chemical and Physical Properties of Molecules

Question 23: What is the molecular formula of ethanol?

A) CH4

B) C2H5OH

C) C6H12O6

D) H2O

Answer: B) C2H5OH

Explanation: The molecular formula of ethanol is C2H5OH.

24. Nomenclature

Question 24: What is the IUPAC name for CH3-CH2-OH?

A) Methanol

B) Ethanol

C) Propanol

D) Isopropanol

Answer: B) Ethanol

Explanation: The IUPAC name for CH3-CH2-OH is ethanol.

25. Functional Group Chemistry

Question 25: Which functional group contains a carbonyl and an amino group?

A) Ester

B) Amine

C) Aldehyde

D) Amide

Answer: D) Amide

Explanation: Amides contain a carbonyl group (C=O) and an amino group (NH2).

Section 1: The Perceptual Ability

26. Apertures

Question 26: Which shape would result from passing a pyramid through a square aperture?

A) Triangle

B) Square

C) Rectangle

D) Circle

Answer: A) Triangle

Explanation: A pyramid would create a triangular shape when passed through a square aperture.

27. View Recognition

Question 27: From the front view, how many faces of a pyramid can be seen?

A) 1

B) 2

C) 3

D) 4

Answer: B) 2

Explanation: From a front view, only the front face and the base of the pyramid are visible.

28. Angle Discrimination

Question 28: What is the measure of each interior angle in a square?

A) 45°

B) 60°

C) 90°

D) 120°

Answer: C) 90°

Explanation: Each interior angle in a square measures 90°.

29. Paper Folding

Question 29: If you fold a square paper diagonally, what shape will you get?

A) Triangle

B) Rectangle

C) Pentagon

D) Circle

Answer: A) Triangle

Explanation: Folding a square paper diagonally will result in a triangle.

30. Cube Counting

Question 30: How many cubes are there in a 2x2x2 cube structure?

A) 4

B) 6

C) 8

D) 12

Answer: C) 8

Explanation: A 2x2x2 cube structure contains 8 individual cubes.

31. 3D Form Development

Question 31: Which 3D shape is formed by revolving a right triangle around one of its legs?

A) Sphere

B) Cylinder

C) Cone

D) Pyramid

Answer: C) Cone

Explanation: Revolving a right triangle around one of its legs will create a cone.

Section 2: The Reading Comprehension

32. Comprehension Skills

Question 32: What is an antonym for the word "benevolent"?

A) Malevolent

B) Generous

C) Kind

D) Compassionate

Answer: A) Malevolent

Explanation: "Malevolent" is the antonym of "benevolent."

33. Critical Thinking Skills

Question 33: Which is a logical fallacy?

A) Ad hominem

B) Deductive reasoning

C) Inductive reasoning

D) Syllogism

Answer: A) Ad hominem

Explanation: Ad hominem is a logical fallacy that attacks the person instead of the argument.

Section 3: The Quantitative Reasoning

34. Numerical Calculations

Question 34: What is 11^2?

A) 11

B) 22

C) 110

D) 121

Answer: D) 121

Explanation: $11^2=121$.

35. Algebra

Question 35: Solve for x: $3x-4=11$

A) 3

B) 4

C) 5

D) 6

Answer: C) 5

Explanation: Solving $3x-4=11$ gives $x=5$.

36. Probability and Statistics

Question 36: What is the probability of drawing an Ace from a standard deck of 52 cards?

A) 1/13

B) 1/52

C) 1/4

D) 1/2

Answer: A) 1/13

Explanation: There are 4 Aces in a deck of 52 cards, so the probability is 4/52=1/13.

37. Geometry

Question 37: What is the sum of the interior angles of a square?

A) 180°

B) 270°

C) 360°

D) 720°

Answer: C) 360°

Explanation: A square has 4 angles each of 90°, totaling 360°.

38. Trigonometry

Question 38: What is the cosine of 0 degrees?

A) 0

B) 1

C) 1221

D) 22

Answer: B) 1

Explanation: $\cos(0)=1$.

Section 4: The Biology

39. Cellular and Molecular Biology

Question 39: What is the main energy molecule of the cell?

A) RNA

B) DNA

C) ATP

D) NADH

Answer: C) ATP

Explanation: ATP is the main energy-carrying molecule in the cell.

40. Diversity of Life

Question 40: What type of organism lacks a nucleus?

A) Eukaryote

B) Virus

C) Prokaryote

D) Fungi

Answer: C) Prokaryote

Explanation: Prokaryotes lack a nucleus.

41. Structure and Functions of Systems

Question 41: What structure in the human body is responsible for gas exchange?

A) Liver

B) Kidney

C) Alveoli

D) Heart

Answer: C) Alveoli

Explanation: Alveoli are responsible for gas exchange in the human respiratory system.

42. Genetics

Question 42: What is a genotype?
A) Physical appearance
B) Genetic makeup
C) Environment
D) Behavior

Answer: B) Genetic makeup

Explanation: A genotype is the genetic makeup of an organism.

43. Evolution, Ecology, and Behavior

Question 43: What term refers to the survival and reproduction of the fittest individuals in a population?
A) Mutation
B) Genetic drift
C) Natural selection
D) Speciation

Answer: C) Natural selection

Explanation: Natural selection refers to the survival and reproduction of the fittest individuals in a population.

Section 5: The General Chemistry

44. States of Matter

Question 44: What state of matter has no definite shape but has a definite volume?
A) Solid
B) Liquid
C) Gas
D) Plasma

Answer: B) Liquid
Explanation: Liquids have a definite volume but no definite shape.

45. Solutions

Question 45: What is the pH of pure water?
A) 5
B) 7
C) 10
D) 14

Answer: B) 7
Explanation: The pH of pure water is 7.

46. Kinetics and Equilibrium

Question 46: What does a catalyst do to a chemical reaction?
A) Speeds it up
B) Slows it down
C) Stops it
D) Changes its products

Answer: A) Speeds it up

Explanation: A catalyst speeds up a chemical reaction without being consumed.

47. Atomic and Molecular Structure

Question 47: What type of bond is formed by the sharing of electrons?

A) Ionic

B) Covalent

C) Metallic

D) Hydrogen

Answer: B) Covalent

Explanation: Covalent bonds are formed by the sharing of electrons.

Section 6: The Organic Chemistry

48. Chemical and Physical Properties of Molecules

Question 48: What is the boiling point of water at sea level in degrees Celsius?

A) 0

B) 50

C) 100

D) 212

Answer: C) 100

Explanation: The boiling point of water at sea level is 100°C.

49. Nomenclature

Question 49: What is the IUPAC name for CH3COOH?

A) Acetone

B) Ethanol

C) Acetic acid

D) Methanol

Answer: C) Acetic acid

Explanation: The IUPAC name for CH3COOH is acetic acid.

50. Functional Group Chemistry

Question 50: What functional group is present in alcohols?

A) Carboxyl

B) Hydroxyl

C) Amino

D) Ketone

Answer: B) Hydroxyl

Explanation: Alcohols contain a hydroxyl ($-OH$) functional group.

Section 1: The Perceptual Ability

51. Apertures

Question 51: What shape would result from passing a cylinder through a circular aperture?

A) Circle

B) Oval

C) Square

D) Triangle

Answer: A) Circle

Explanation: A cylinder would create a circular shape when passed through a circular aperture.

52. View Recognition

Question 52: What shape will you see when viewing a cube from above?

A) Square

B) Rectangle

C) Triangle

D) Hexagon

Answer: A) Square

Explanation: From an overhead view, a cube appears as a square.

53. Angle Discrimination

Question 53: What is the sum of the interior angles in a pentagon?

A) 90°

B) 180°

C) 360°

D) 540°

Answer: D) 540°

Explanation: Sum of Interior Angles in a Pentagon = (n-2)× 180°= 3× 180°= 540°.

54. Paper Folding

Question 54: If you fold a rectangle paper in half along its length, what shape will you get?

A) Square

B) Rectangle

C) Triangle

D) Trapezoid

Answer: B) Rectangle

Explanation: Folding a rectangle in half along its length will still result in a rectangle, albeit a smaller one.

55. Cube Counting

Question 55: How many faces are visible when viewing a cube from one corner?

A) 1

B) 2

C) 3

D) 4

Answer: C) 3

Explanation: When viewing a cube from one corner, three faces are visible.

56. 3D Form Development

Question 56: What 3D shape is formed when a rectangle is rotated around one of its sides?

A) Cone

B) Cylinder

C) Sphere

D) Cube

Answer: B) Cylinder

Explanation: When a rectangle is rotated around one of its sides, a cylinder is formed.

Section 2: The Reading Comprehension

57. Comprehension Skills

Question 57: What is a synonym for the word "altruistic"?
A) Selfish
B) Benevolent
C) Malevolent
D) Apathetic

Answer: B) Benevolent

Explanation: "Benevolent" is a synonym for "altruistic."

58. Critical Thinking Skills

Question 58: Which is an example of a post hoc fallacy?
A) Slippery slope
B) Ad hominem
C) Circular reasoning
D) Correlation implies causation

Answer: D) Correlation implies causation

Explanation: A post hoc fallacy occurs when it's assumed that correlation implies causation.

Section 3: The Quantitative Reasoning

59. Numerical Calculations

Question 59: What is 7^2?

A) 14

B) 49

C) 28

D) 64

Answer: B) 49

Explanation: $7^2=49$.

60. Algebra

Question 60: Solve for x: $5x+3=28$

A) 4

B) 5

C) 6

D) 7

Answer: B) 5

Explanation: Solving $5x+3=28$ gives $x=5$.

61. Probability and Statistics

Question 61: If you roll a standard six-sided die twice, what is the probability of getting two 6s?

A) 1/6

B) 1/12

C) 1/36

D) 1/72

Answer: C) 1/36

Explanation: When rolling a die twice, each roll is independent. The probability of getting a 6 on a single roll is 1/6, so the probability of getting two 6s is (1/6) * (1/6) = 1/36.

62. Geometry

Question 62: What is the area of a circle with a radius of 7 cm?
A) 49π cm²
B) 14π cm²
C) 21π cm²
D) 28π cm²

Answer: A) 49π cm²
Explanation: The area of a circle is πr^2, which would be 49π cm² for a radius of 7 cm.

63. Trigonometry

Question 63: What is the sine of 90 degrees?
A) 0
B) 1
C) 0.5
D) 2222

Answer: B) 1
Explanation: $\sin(90°)=1$.

Section 4: The Biology

64. Cellular and Molecular Biology

Question 64: What organelle is responsible for photosynthesis?

A) Mitochondria

B) Chloroplast

C) Nucleus

D) Ribosome

Answer: B) Chloroplast

Explanation: Chloroplasts are responsible for photosynthesis.

65. Diversity of Life

Question 65: What kingdom includes mushrooms?

A) Animalia

B) Plantae

C) Fungi

D) Protista

Answer: C) Fungi

Explanation: Mushrooms belong to the kingdom Fungi.

66. Structure and Functions of Systems

Question 66: What organ produces insulin?

A) Liver

B) Pancreas

C) Kidneys

D) Heart

Answer: B) Pancreas

Explanation: The pancreas produces insulin.

67. Genetics

Question 67: What are the building blocks of DNA?

A) Amino acids

B) Nucleotides

C) Fatty acids

D) Carbohydrates

Answer: B) Nucleotides

Explanation: Nucleotides are the building blocks of DNA.

68. Evolution, Ecology, and Behavior

Question 68: What is the primary role of decomposers in an ecosystem?

A) Predation

B) Photosynthesis

C) Nutrient recycling

D) Pollination

Answer: C) Nutrient recycling

Explanation: Decomposers play a primary role in recycling nutrients within an ecosystem.

Section 5: The General Chemistry

69. States of Matter

Question 69: What is the process of a gas turning into a liquid?

A) Condensation

B) Sublimation

C) Evaporation

D) Fusion

Answer: A) Condensation

Explanation: The process of a gas turning into a liquid is called condensation.

70. Solutions

Question 70: What is the solvent in a sugar water solution?

A) Sugar

B) Water

C) Neither

D) Both

Answer: B) Water

Explanation: In a sugar water solution, water is the solvent.

71. Kinetics and Equilibrium

Question 71: What is the equilibrium constant for a reaction that has reached equilibrium?

A) 0

B) 1

C) Less than 1

D) Greater than 1

Answer: D) Greater than 1

Explanation: The equilibrium constant for a reaction that has reached equilibrium can be greater than 1, depending on the reaction.

72. Atomic and Molecular Structure

Question 72: How many electrons does an atom of helium have?

A) 1

B) 2

C) 3

D) 4

Answer: B) 2

Explanation: An atom of helium has 2 electrons.

Section 6: The Organic Chemistry

73. Chemical and Physical Properties of Molecules

Question 73: What is the melting point of ice in Fahrenheit?

A) 0

B) 32

C) 100

D) 212

Answer: B) 32

Explanation: The melting point of ice in Fahrenheit is 32°F.

74. Nomenclature

Question 74: What is the IUPAC name for CH_4?

A) Ethane

B) Methane

C) Propane

D) Butane

Answer: B) Methane

Explanation: The IUPAC name for CH4 is methane.

75. Functional Group Chemistry

Question 75: What functional group is present in carboxylic acids?

A) Amino

B) Hydroxyl

C) Carbonyl

D) Carboxyl

Answer: D) Carboxyl

Explanation: Carboxylic acids contain a carboxyl ($-COOH$) functional group.

Section 1: The Perceptual Ability

76. Apertures

Question 76: What shape would result from passing a square through a circular aperture?

A) Circle

B) Square

C) Oval

D) Trapezoid

Answer: B) Square

Explanation: A square would remain square when passed through a circular aperture.

77. View Recognition

Question 77: What shape will you see when viewing a pyramid from above?

A) Triangle

B) Square

C) Circle

D) Hexagon

Answer: B) Square

Explanation: From an overhead view, a pyramid typically appears as a square.

78. Angle Discrimination

Question 78: What is the measure of each interior angle in an hexagon?

A) 30°

B) 45°

C) 60°

D) 120°

Answer: C) 60°

Explanation: Each angle in an hexagon measures 120°.

79. Paper Folding

Question 79: If you fold a square paper diagonally, what shape will result?

A) Triangle

B) Rectangle

C) Square

D) Trapezoid

Answer: A) Triangle

Explanation: Folding a square paper diagonally will result in a triangle.

80. Cube Counting

Question 80: How many edges does a cube have?

A) 8

B) 12

C) 16

D) 20

Answer: B) 12

Explanation: A cube has 12 edges.

81. 3D Form Development

Question 81: What 3D shape is formed when a right triangle is rotated about one of its legs?

A) Cone

B) Cylinder

C) Sphere

D) Pyramid

Answer: A) Cone

Explanation: Rotating a right triangle about one of its legs will form a cone.

Section 2: The Reading Comprehension

82. Comprehension Skills

Question 82: What is the antonym of the word "benevolent"?

A) Malevolent

B) Kind

C) Charitable

D) Generous

Answer: A) Malevolent

Explanation: "Malevolent" is the antonym of "benevolent."

83. Critical Thinking Skills

Question 83: Which of these is a straw man fallacy?

A) Slippery slope

B) Ad hominem

C) Circular reasoning

D) Misrepresenting an argument

Answer: D) Misrepresenting an argument

Explanation: A straw man fallacy occurs when an argument is misrepresented to make it easier to attack.

Section 3: The Quantitative Reasoning

84. Numerical Calculations

Question 84: What is 13^2?

A) 13

B) 26

C) 130

D) 169

Answer: D) 169

Explanation: $13^2 = 169$.

85. Algebra

Question 85: Solve for x: $3x-4=14$

A) 2

B) 3

C) 5

D) 6

Answer: D) 6

Explanation: Solving $3x-4=14$ gives $x=6$.

86. Probability and Statistics

Question 86: What is the probability of flipping heads on a standard coin?

A) 1/2

B) 1/3

C) 1/4

D) 1/6

Answer: A) 1/2

Explanation: The probability of flipping heads on a standard coin is 1/2.

87. Geometry

Question 87: What is the area of a square with sides of 8 cm?

A) 32 cm²

B) 64 cm²

C) 128 cm²

D) 256 cm²

Answer: B) 64 cm²

Explanation: The area of a square with sides of 8 cm is $8 \times 8 = 64$ cm².

88. Trigonometry

Question 88: What is the cosine of 0 degrees?

A) 0

B) 1

C) 0.5

D) 2222

Answer: B) 1

Explanation: cos(0°)=1.

Section 4: The Biology

89. Cellular and Molecular Biology

Question 89: Which molecule serves as the energy currency of the cell?

A) Glucose

B) ATP

C) Protein

D) DNA

Answer: B) ATP

Explanation: ATP serves as the energy currency of the cell.

90. Diversity of Life

Question 90: Which kingdom do bacteria belong to?

A) Animalia

B) Plantae

C) Fungi

D) Prokaryotae

Answer: D) Prokaryotae

Explanation: Bacteria belong to the kingdom Prokaryotae, also known as Monera.

91. Structure and Functions of Systems

Question 91: What is the main function of red blood cells?

A) Immunity

B) Oxygen transport

C) Clotting

D) Filtering toxins

Answer: B) Oxygen transport

Explanation: The main function of red blood cells is to transport oxygen.

92. Genetics

Question 92: What is a gene made up of?

A) Proteins

B) Carbohydrates

C) Lipids

D) DNA

Answer: D) DNA

Explanation: A gene is made up of DNA.

93. Evolution, Ecology, and Behavior

Question 93: What do herbivores primarily eat?

A) Meat

B) Plants

C) Fungi

D) Both meat and plants

Answer: B) Plants

Explanation: Herbivores primarily eat plants.

Section 5: The General Chemistry

94. States of Matter

Question 94: What state of matter has a fixed shape and volume?

A) Solid

B) Liquid

C) Gas

D) Plasma

Answer: A) Solid

Explanation: Solids have a fixed shape and volume.

95. Solutions

Question 95: What does it mean if a solution is "saturated"?

A) It cannot dissolve more solute

B) It can dissolve more solute

C) It is highly reactive

D) It is colorless

Answer: A) It cannot dissolve more solute

Explanation: A "saturated" solution cannot dissolve any more solute.

96. Kinetics and Equilibrium

Question 96: What does it mean if the rate constant (k) of a reaction is high?

A) Slow reaction

B) Fast reaction

C) Equilibrium is not reached

D) Reaction is irreversible

Answer: B) Fast reaction

Explanation: A high rate constant (k) indicates a fast reaction.

97. Atomic and Molecular Structure

Question 97: What is the atomic number of hydrogen?

A) 0

B) 1

C) 2

D) 3

Answer: B) 1

Explanation: The atomic number of hydrogen is 1.

Section 6: The Organic Chemistry

98. Chemical and Physical Properties of Molecules

Question 98: What is the boiling point of water in Celsius?

A) 0

B) 50

C) 100

D) 212

Answer: C) 100

Explanation: The boiling point of water in Celsius is 100°C.

99. Nomenclature

Question 99: What is the IUPAC name for C_2H_6?

A) Ethane

B) Methane

C) Propane

D) Butane

Answer: A) Ethane

Explanation: The IUPAC name for C_2H_6 is ethane.

100. Functional Group Chemistry

Question 100: What functional group is present in alcohols?

A) Amino

B) Hydroxyl

C) Carbonyl

D) Carboxyl

Answer: B) Hydroxyl

Explanation: Alcohols contain a hydroxyl $(-OH)$ functional group.

FULL-LENGTH PRACTICE TEST 2

Section 1: The Perceptual Ability

101. Apertures

Question 101: Which shape would result if a circle passes through a square aperture?
A) Circle
B) Square
C) Oval
D) Trapezoid

Answer: A) Circle
Explanation: A circle would remain a circle when passed through a square aperture.

102. View Recognition

Question 102: What shape would a cone look like when viewed from the side?
A) Triangle
B) Rectangle
C) Oval
D) Circle

Answer: A) Triangle

Explanation: From a side view, a cone would look like a triangle.

103. Angle Discrimination

Question 103: What is the sum of interior angles in a hexagon?

A) 540°

B) 720°

C) 900°

D) 1080°

Answer: B) 720°

Explanation: The sum of interior angles in a hexagon is 720°.

104. Paper Folding

Question 104: What shape will result if you fold a rectangular paper in half along its length?

A) Triangle

B) Square

C) Rectangle

D) Parallelogram

Answer: C) Rectangle

Explanation: Folding a rectangular paper in half along its length will result in another rectangle.

105. Cube Counting

Question 105: How many faces does a cube have?

A) 4

B) 6
C) 8
D) 12

Answer: B) 6
Explanation: A cube has 6 faces.

106. 3D Form Development

Question 106: What shape will be formed when you rotate a rectangle about its longer side?
A) Cylinder
B) Cone
C) Sphere
D) Pyramid

Answer: A) Cylinder
Explanation: Rotating a rectangle about its longer side will form a cylinder.

Section 2: The Reading Comprehension

107. Comprehension Skills

Question 107: What is the synonym of "malevolent"?
A) Benevolent
B) Evil
C) Kind
D) Generous

Answer: B) Evil
Explanation: "Evil" is a synonym for "malevolent."

108. Critical Thinking Skills

Question 108: What is the opposite of deductive reasoning?

A) Abductive reasoning

B) Inductive reasoning

C) Circumstantial reasoning

D) Syllogistic reasoning

Answer: B) Inductive reasoning

Explanation: The opposite of deductive reasoning is inductive reasoning.

Section 3: The Quantitative Reasoning

109. Numerical Calculations

Question 109: What is 9^3?

A) 9

B) 27

C) 81

D) 729

Answer: D) 729

Explanation: 9^3=729.

110. Algebra

Question 110: Solve for y: $2y+3=9$

A) 1

B) 2

C) 3
D) 4

Answer: C) 3
Explanation: Solving $2y+3=9$ gives $y=3$.

111. Probability and Statistics

Question 111: What is the mean of the numbers 1, 2, and 3?
A) 1
B) 2
C) 3
D) 6

Answer: B) 2
Explanation: The mean of the numbers 1, 2, and 3 is 2.

112. Geometry

Question 112: What is the perimeter of a square with sides of 5 cm?
A) 15 cm
B) 20 cm
C) 25 cm
D) 30 cm

Answer: B) 20 cm
Explanation: The perimeter of a square with sides of 5 cm is $4\times5=20$ cm.

113. Trigonometry

Question 113: What is the sine of 90 degrees?
A) 0

B) 1

C) 1221

D) 2222

Answer: B) 1

Explanation: $\sin(90°)=1$.

Section 4: The Biology

114. Cellular and Molecular Biology

Question 114: What is the primary function of the mitochondria?

A) Photosynthesis

B) Energy production

C) Protein synthesis

D) Cell division

Answer: B) Energy production

Explanation: The primary function of the mitochondria is energy production.

115. Diversity of Life

Question 115: What is the scientific name for humans?

A) Homo erectus

B) Homo neanderthalensis

C) Homo sapiens

D) Homo habilis

Answer: C) Homo sapiens

Explanation: The scientific name for humans is Homo sapiens.

116. Structure and Functions of Systems

Question 116: What is the main function of the nervous system?

A) Respiration

B) Digestion

C) Communication and coordination

D) Immunity

Answer: C) Communication and coordination

Explanation: The main function of the nervous system is communication and coordination.

117. Genetics

Question 117: What is the DNA base pair for adenine?

A) Thymine

B) Guanine

C) Cytosine

D) Uracil

Answer: A) Thymine

Explanation: Adenine pairs with thymine in DNA.

118. Evolution, Ecology, and Behavior

Question 118: What type of mimicry is displayed when a harmless species mimics a harmful species?

A) Batesian mimicry

B) Müllerian mimicry

C) Mertensian mimicry

D) Automimicry

Answer: A) Batesian mimicry

Explanation: When a harmless species mimics a harmful species, it is called Batesian mimicry.

Section 5: The General Chemistry

119. States of Matter

Question 119: What is the process of a liquid turning into a gas called?

A) Freezing

B) Condensation

C) Evaporation

D) Sublimation

Answer: C) Evaporation

Explanation: The process of a liquid turning into a gas is called evaporation.

120. Solutions

Question 120: What is the solvent in a sugar-water solution?

A) Sugar

B) Water

C) Neither

D) Both

Answer: B) Water

Explanation: In a sugar-water solution, water is the solvent.

121. Kinetics and Equilibrium

Question 121: At what point is a chemical reaction in equilibrium?

A) When reactants are fully converted to products

B) When the rate of the forward reaction equals the rate of the reverse reaction

C) When all reactants and products are gone

D) When the reaction is completed quickly

Answer: B) When the rate of the forward reaction equals the rate of the reverse reaction

Explanation: A chemical reaction is in equilibrium when the rate of the forward reaction equals the rate of the reverse reaction.

122. Atomic and Molecular Structure

Question 122: Which element has the atomic number 2?

A) Hydrogen

B) Helium

C) Lithium

D) Beryllium

Answer: B) Helium

Explanation: The element with the atomic number 2 is helium.

Section 6: The Organic Chemistry

123. Chemical and Physical Properties of Molecules

Question 123: What type of bond is found in a water molecule?

A) Ionic

B) Covalent

C) Metallic

D) Van der Waals

Answer: B) Covalent

Explanation: A covalent bond is found in a water molecule.

124. Nomenclature

Question 124: What is the IUPAC name for C_4H_{10}?

A) Methane

B) Ethane

C) Butane

D) Propane

Answer: C) Butane

Explanation: The IUPAC name for C_4H_{10} is butane.

125. Functional Group Chemistry

Question 125: What functional group is present in ketones?

A) Amino

B) Hydroxyl

C) Carbonyl

D) Carboxyl

Answer: C) Carbonyl

Explanation: Ketones contain a carbonyl (C=O) functional group.

Section 1: The Perceptual Ability

126. Apertures

Question 126: What shape would result if a square passes through a circular aperture?

A) Circle

B) Square

C) Oval

D) Rectangle

Answer: B) Square

Explanation: A square would remain a square when passed through a circular aperture.

127. View Recognition

Question 127: What shape would a sphere look like when viewed from the top?

A) Circle

B) Ellipse

C) Square

D) Triangle

Answer: A) Circle

Explanation: From a top view, a sphere would look like a circle.

128. Angle Discrimination

Question 128: What is the measure of each interior angle in an equilateral triangle?

A) 45°

B) 60°

C) 90°

D) 120°

Answer: B) 60°

Explanation: Each interior angle in an equilateral triangle is 60°.

129. Paper Folding

Question 129: What shape will result if you fold a square paper diagonally?

A) Triangle

B) Rectangle

C) Square

D) Parallelogram

Answer: A) Triangle

Explanation: Folding a square paper diagonally will result in a triangle.

130. Cube Counting

Question 130: How many vertices does a cube have?

A) 4

B) 6

C) 8

D) 12

Answer: C) 8

Explanation: A cube has 8 vertices.

131. 3D Form Development

Question 131: What shape will be formed when you rotate a triangle about its base?

A) Cone

B) Cylinder

C) Sphere

D) Pyramid

Answer: A) Cone

Explanation: Rotating a triangle about its base will form a cone.

Section 2: The Reading Comprehension

132. Comprehension Skills

Question 132: What is the antonym of "prolific"?
A) Fertile
B) Barren
C) Abundant
D) Overflowing

Answer: B) Barren

Explanation: "Barren" is the antonym of "prolific."

133. Critical Thinking Skills

Question 133: Which type of reasoning starts with a generalization and moves towards a specific conclusion?
A) Deductive
B) Inductive
C) Abductive
D) Analogical

Answer: A) Deductive

Explanation: Deductive reasoning starts with a generalization and moves towards a specific conclusion.

Section 3: The Quantitative Reasoning

134. Numerical Calculations

Question 134: What is 7^2?

A) 14

B) 49

C) 28

D) 64

Answer: B) 49

Explanation: $7^2=49$.

135. Algebra

Question 135: Solve for x: $5x-10=20$

A) 2

B) 4

C) 6

D) 8

Answer: C) 6

Explanation: Solving $5x-10=20$ gives $x=6$.

136. Probability and Statistics

Question 136: What is the median of the numbers 3, 7, 5, 9, and 4?

A) 5

B) 6

C) 7

D) 8

Answer: A) 5

Explanation: When arranged in ascending order (3, 4, 5, 7, 9), the median is 5.

137. Geometry

Question 137: What is the area of a circle with a radius of 3 cm? (Use π=3.14)

A) 9.42 cm²

B) 18.84 cm²

C) 28.26 cm²

D) 37.68 cm²

Answer: C) 28.26 cm²

Explanation: The area of a circle is πr^2, which in this case is 3.14×3×3=28.26 3.14×3×3=28.26 cm².

138. Trigonometry

Question 138: What is the cosine of 0 degrees?

A) 0

B) 1

C) 1/2

D) -1

Answer: B) 1

Explanation: cos(0°)=1.

Section 4: The Biology

139. Cellular and Molecular Biology

Question 139: What is the site of protein synthesis in a cell?

A) Mitochondria

B) Ribosome

C) Nucleus

D) Golgi apparatus

Answer: B) Ribosome

Explanation: The ribosome is the site of protein synthesis in a cell.

140. Diversity of Life

Question 140: What is the most abundant gas in Earth's atmosphere?

A) Oxygen

B) Carbon dioxide

C) Nitrogen

D) Hydrogen

Answer: C) Nitrogen

Explanation: Nitrogen is the most abundant gas in Earth's atmosphere.

141. Structure and Functions of Systems

Question 141: What is the function of white blood cells?

A) Transport oxygen

B) Clot blood

C) Fight infection

D) Regulate temperature

Answer: C) Fight infection

Explanation: White blood cells are responsible for fighting infections.

142. Genetics

Question 142: What do you call the physical expression of a genetic trait?

A) Genotype

B) Phenotype

C) Allele

D) Chromosome

Answer: B) Phenotype

Explanation: The physical expression of a genetic trait is called the phenotype.

143. Evolution, Ecology, and Behavior

Question 143: What do you call a relationship where both species benefit?

A) Parasitism

B) Mutualism

C) Commensalism

D) Predation

Answer: B) Mutualism

Explanation: A relationship where both species benefit is called mutualism.

Section 5: The General Chemistry

144. States of Matter

Question 144: What is the process of a solid turning into a liquid called?

A) Melting

B) Freezing

C) Evaporation

D) Condensation

Answer: A) Melting

Explanation: The process of a solid turning into a liquid is called melting.

145. Solutions

Question 145: What is the solute in a sugar-water solution?

A) Sugar

B) Water

C) Neither

D) Both

Answer: A) Sugar

Explanation: In a sugar-water solution, sugar is the solute.

146. Kinetics and Equilibrium

Question 146: What is the activation energy of a chemical reaction?

A) The energy needed to break bonds in reactants

B) The energy released during the reaction

C) The total energy in the system

D) The energy of the products

Answer: A) The energy needed to break bonds in reactants

Explanation: The activation energy is the energy required to break bonds in reactants and initiate a chemical reaction.

147. Atomic and Molecular Structure

Question 147: Which element has the atomic number 3?

A) Hydrogen

B) Helium

C) Lithium

D) Beryllium

Answer: C) Lithium

Explanation: The element with the atomic number 3 is lithium.

Section 6: The Organic Chemistry

148. Chemical and Physical Properties of Molecules

Question 148: What type of bond is found in salt (NaCl)?

A) Covalent

B) Ionic

C) Metallic

D) Hydrogen

Answer: B) Ionic

Explanation: An ionic bond is found in salt (NaCl).

149. Nomenclature

Question 149: What is the IUPAC name for C5H12C5H12?

A) Methane

B) Ethane

C) Butane

D) Pentane

Answer: D) Pentane

Explanation: The IUPAC name for C5H12C5H12 is pentane.

150. Functional Group Chemistry

Question 150: What functional group is present in alcohols?

A) Amino

B) Hydroxyl

C) Carbonyl

D) Carboxyl

Answer: B) Hydroxyl

Explanation: Alcohols contain a hydroxyl (OHOH) functional group.

Section 1: The Perceptual Ability

151. Apertures

Question 151: What shape would result if a rectangle passes through a circular aperture?

A) Circle

B) Rectangle

C) Oval

D) Square

Answer: B) Rectangle

Explanation: A rectangle would remain a rectangle when passed through a circular aperture.

152. View Recognition

Question 152: What shape would a cylinder look like when viewed from the side?

A) Circle

B) Rectangle

C) Square

D) Triangle

Answer: B) Rectangle

Explanation: From a side view, a cylinder would look like a rectangle.

153. Angle Discrimination

Question 153: What is the measure of each interior angle in a square?

A) 45°

B) 90°

C) 120°

D) 60°

Answer: B) 90°

Explanation: Each interior angle in a square is 90°.

154. Paper Folding

Question 154: What shape will result if you fold a rectangular paper in half vertically?

A) Square

B) Rectangle

C) Triangle

D) Parallelogram

Answer: B) Rectangle

Explanation: Folding a rectangular paper in half vertically will result in another rectangle.

155. Cube Counting

Question 155: How many faces does a cube have?

A) 4

B) 6

C) 8

D) 12

Answer: B) 6

Explanation: A cube has 6 faces.

156. 3D Form Development

Question 156: What shape will be formed when you rotate a rectangle about its longer side?

A) Cone

B) Cylinder

C) Sphere

D) Pyramid

Answer: B) Cylinder

Explanation: Rotating a rectangle about its longer side will form a cylinder.

Section 2: The Reading Comprehension

157. Comprehension Skills

Question 157: What is the synonym of "benevolent"?

A) Malevolent

B) Kind

C) Selfish

D) Indifferent

Answer: B) Kind

Explanation: "Kind" is a synonym for "benevolent."

158. Critical Thinking Skills

Question 158: Which type of reasoning uses specific observations to make general conclusions?
A) Deductive
B) Inductive
C) Abductive
D) Analogical

Answer: B) Inductive

Explanation: Inductive reasoning uses specific observations to make general conclusions.

Section 3: The Quantitative Reasoning

159. Numerical Calculations

Question 159: What is 11^3?
A) 11
B) 33
C) 121
D) 1331

Answer: D) 1331

Explanation: $11^3 = 1331$.

160. Algebra

Question 160: Solve for x: $3x+4=19$

A) 3

B) 5

C) 7

D) 9

Answer: B) 5

Explanation: Solving $3x+4=19$ gives $x=5$.

161. Probability and Statistics

Question 161: What is the mode of the numbers 4, 5, 6, 4, 7?

A) 4

B) 5

C) 6

D) 7

Answer: A) 4

Explanation: The mode is the number that appears most frequently, which is 4 in this set.

162. Geometry

Question 162: What is the volume of a cube with a side length of 2 cm?

A) 4 cm³

B) 6 cm³

C) 8 cm³

D) 16 cm³

Answer: C) 8 cm³

Explanation: The volume of a cube is s^3, which in this case is $2^3=8$ cm³.

163. Trigonometry

Question 163: What is the sine of 30 degrees?

A) 0

B) 1

C) 1/2

D) -1

Answer: C) 1/2

Explanation: sin(30°)=1/2.

Section 4: The Biology

164. Cellular and Molecular Biology

Question 164: What molecule stores genetic information in a cell?

A) DNA

B) RNA

C) ATP

D) Enzyme

Answer: A) DNA

Explanation: DNA stores genetic information in a cell.

165. Diversity of Life

Question 165: What type of organism performs photosynthesis?

A) Bacteria

B) Animals

C) Plants

D) Fungi

Answer: C) Plants

Explanation: Plants perform photosynthesis.

166. Structure and Functions of Systems

Question 166: What is the main function of the heart?

A) Digestion

B) Circulation

C) Respiration

D) Regulation

Answer: B) Circulation

Explanation: The main function of the heart is to circulate blood throughout the body.

167. Genetics

Question 167: What is a set of three nucleotides that codes

continue from 167ChatGPT

for a specific amino acid?

A) Codon

B) Allele

C) Exon

D) Intron

Answer: A) Codon

Explanation: A codon is a set of three nucleotides that codes for a specific amino acid.

168. Evolution, Ecology, and Behavior

Question 168: Which of the following factors would most directly affect the carrying capacity of an ecosystem?
A) Mutation rate
B) Available resources
C) Species diversity
D) Temperature variation

Answer: B) Available resources

Explanation: The carrying capacity of an ecosystem is most directly affected by the availability of resources.

Section 5: The General Chemistry

169. States of Matter

Question 169: What state of matter has definite shape and volume?
A) Gas
B) Liquid
C) Solid
D) Plasma

Answer: C) Solid

Explanation: Solids have definite shape and volume.

170. Solutions

Question 170: What is the solvent in a sugar-water solution?

A) Sugar

B) Water

C) Both

D) None

Answer: B) Water

Explanation: In a sugar-water solution, water is the solvent.

171. Kinetics and Equilibrium

Question 171: What factor would increase the rate of a chemical reaction?

A) Decreasing temperature

B) Increasing concentration of reactants

C) Decreasing pressure

D) Adding a catalyst in lesser amount

Answer: B) Increasing concentration of reactants

Explanation: Increasing the concentration of reactants generally increases the rate of a chemical reaction.

172. Atomic and Molecular Structure

Question 172: What is the atomic number of an element that has 6 protons?

A) 4

B) 6

C) 8

D) 12

Answer: B) 6

Explanation: The atomic number is equal to the number of protons, so it would be 6.

Section 6: The Organic Chemistry

173. Chemical and Physical Properties of Molecules

Question 173: Which of the following is a polar molecule?
A) CH_4
B) O_2
C) H_2O
D) N_2

Answer: C) H_2O

Explanation: H_2O is a polar molecule due to its bent shape and the difference in electronegativity between oxygen and hydrogen.

174. Nomenclature

Question 174: What is the prefix used to indicate six carbon atoms in an alkane?
A) Meth-
B) Eth-
C) Prop-
D) Hex-

Answer: D) Hex-

Explanation: The prefix "Hex-" is used to indicate an alkane with six carbon atoms.

175. Functional Group Chemistry

Question 175: What functional group is found in alcohols?

A) -COOH

B) -NH2

C) -OH

D) -C=O

Answer: C) -OH

Explanation: Alcohols contain the -OH functional group.

Section 1: The Perceptual Ability

176. Apertures

Question 176: Which shape would fit perfectly into a pentagon-shaped hole?

A) Square

B) Triangle

C) Pentagon

D) Hexagon

Answer: C) Pentagon

Explanation: A pentagon would fit perfectly into a pentagon-shaped hole.

177. View Recognition

Question 177: If you look at a cube from the top, how many faces will be visible?

A) 1

B) 2

C) 3

D) 4

Answer: A) 1

Explanation: When looking at a cube from the top, only the top face is visible.

178. Angle Discrimination

Question 178: What is the smallest angle in an isosceles right triangle?

A) 30 degrees

B) 45 degrees

C) 90 degrees

D) 60 degrees

Answer: B) 45 degrees

Explanation: In an isosceles right triangle, the smallest angle is 45 degrees.

179. Paper Folding

Question 179: If a square paper is folded in half, what shape will result?

A) Rectangle

B) Square

C) Triangle

D) Rhombus

Answer: A) Rectangle

Explanation: A square folded in half will form a rectangle.

180. Cube Counting

Question 180: How many cubes make up a 3x3x3 Rubik's Cube?

A) 9

B) 18

C) 27

D) 36

Answer: C) 27

Explanation: A 3x3x3 Rubik's Cube consists of 27 smaller cubes.

181. 3D Form Development

Question 181: If a sphere is cut into two equal halves, what 3D shape results?

A) Cone

B) Hemisphere

C) Cylinder

D) Cube

Answer: B) Hemisphere

Explanation: Cutting a sphere into two equal halves creates hemispheres.

Section 2: The Reading Comprehension

182. Comprehension Skills

Question 182: Which of the following best describes the main idea?

A) Summary

B) Details

C) Theme

D) Conclusion

Answer: C) Theme

Explanation: The main idea is best described as the theme of a passage.

183. Critical Thinking Skills

Question 183: Which of the following is NOT a logical fallacy?

A) Ad Hominem

B) Strawman

C) Slippery Slope

D) Deductive Reasoning

Answer: D) Deductive Reasoning

Explanation: Deductive reasoning is not a logical fallacy; it's a method of logical argument.

Section 3: The Quantitative Reasoning

184. Numerical Calculations

Question 184: What is 20% of 200?

A) 20

B) 40

C) 50

D) 60

Answer: B) 40

Explanation: 20% of 200 is 40.

185. Algebra

Question 185: If $x+4=12$, what is x?

A) 6

B) 7

C) 8

D) 9

Answer: C) 8

Explanation: If $x+4=12$, then �$=8x=8$.

186. Probability and Statistics

Question 186: In a single toss of a fair six-sided die, what is the probability of rolling a 3?

A) 1/2

B) 1/4

C) 1/6

D) 1/8

Answer: C) 1/6

Explanation: There is 1 favorable outcome (rolling a 3) out of 6 possible outcomes, so the probability is 1/6.

187. Geometry

Question 187: What is the sum of the interior angles of a pentagon?

A) 90 degrees

B) 180 degrees

C) 540 degrees

D) 360 degrees

Answer: C) 540 degrees

Explanation: The sum of the interior angles of a pentagon is always 540 degrees.

188. Trigonometry

Question 188: What is the sine of 0 degrees?

A) 0

B) 0.5

C) 1

D) Undefined

Answer: A) 0

Explanation: The sine of 0 degrees is 0.

Section 4: The Biology

189. Cellular and Molecular Biology

Question 189: What organelle is responsible for ATP production?

A) Ribosome

B) Mitochondria

C) Nucleus

D) Endoplasmic Reticulum

Answer: B) Mitochondria

Explanation: The mitochondria are responsible for ATP production.

190. Diversity of Life

Question 190: Which of the following organisms is unicellular?

A) Human

B) Amoeba

C) Tree

D) Frog

Answer: B) Amoeba

Explanation: An amoeba is a unicellular organism.

191. Structure and Functions of Systems

Question 191: What is the main function of the respiratory system?

A) Digestion

B) Circulation

C) Gas exchange

D) Excretion

Answer: C) Gas exchange

Explanation: The main function of the respiratory system is gas exchange.

192. Genetics

Question 192: What does a Punnett Square predict?

A) Age

B) Physical features

C) Genetic outcomes

D) IQ levels

Answer: C) Genetic outcomes

Explanation: A Punnett Square is used to predict the possible genetic outcomes of offspring.

193. Evolution, Ecology, and Behavior

Question 193: Which of the following is an example of a behavioral adaptation?

A) Webbed feet

B) Migration

C) Fur color

D) Long neck

Answer: B) Migration

Explanation: Migration is a behavioral adaptation to environmental conditions.

Section 5: The General Chemistry

194. States of Matter

Question 194: Which state of matter takes the shape of its container but has a fixed volume?
A) Solid
B) Liquid
C) Gas
D) Plasma

Answer: B) Liquid

Explanation: Liquids take the shape of their container but have a fixed volume.

195. Solutions

Question 195: What is the solute in a salt-water solution?
A) Salt
B) Water
C) Both
D) None

Answer: A) Salt

Explanation: In a salt-water solution, salt is the solute.

196. Kinetics and Equilibrium

Question 196: What is the equilibrium constant *K* for a reaction that favors the products?

A) $K<1$

B) $K=1$

C) $K>1$

D) $K=0$

Answer: C) $K>1$

Explanation: For a reaction that favors the products, the equilibrium constant *K* would be greater than 1.

197. Atomic and Molecular Structure

Question 197: How many electrons does a neutral atom of Helium have?

A) 1

B) 2

C) 3

D) 4

Answer: B) 2

Explanation: A neutral atom of Helium has 2 electrons, which equals the number of protons.

Section 6: The Organic Chemistry

198. Chemical and Physical Properties of Molecules

Question 198: Which of the following molecules is nonpolar?

A) CH_4

B) H_2O

C) NH3

D) HCl

Answer: A) CH4

Explanation: CH4 is nonpolar because it has a symmetrical arrangement of atoms and no net dipole moment.

199. Nomenclature

Question 199: What is the IUPAC name for CH_3CH_2OH?

A) Methanol

B) Ethanol

C) Propanol

D) Butanol

Answer: B) Ethanol

Explanation: The IUPAC name for CH_3CH_2OH is Ethanol.

200. Functional Group Chemistry

Question 200: What functional group is found in ketones?

A) -COOH

B) -NH2

C) -OH

D) -C=O

Answer: D) -C=O

Explanation: Ketones contain the -C=O functional group.

TEST-TAKING STRATEGIES

Mastering the content is only one part of your journey to success in the Dental Admission Test (DAT) Exam. Equally important are the strategies you employ on test day and your ability to overcome the challenges of test anxiety. In this chapter, we'll explore effective test-taking strategies and offer guidance on keeping anxiety at bay.

Preparing for Test Day

- A successful test day begins with thorough preparation. Learn what to do in the days leading up to the DAT Exam to ensure you're ready and confident.

Time Management Techniques

- Effective time management is essential during the DAT Exam. Explore strategies for allocating your time wisely and ensuring you have ample time to complete each section.

Question Analysis and Approach

- Discover how to dissect DAT questions effectively, ensuring you understand what is being asked and how to approach each question strategically.

- Learn techniques for eliminating answer choices and making informed

145

decisions.

Navigating Multiple-Choice Questions

- Multiple-choice questions are a common format in the DAT Exam. Find out how to tackle these questions with confidence, even when you're uncertain about the answer.

Strategies for Different Sections

- Each section of the DAT Exam may require unique strategies. We'll explore specific approaches for the Perceptual Ability, Reading Comprehension, Quantitative Reasoning, Biology, General Chemistry, and Organic Chemistry sections.

Managing Test Anxiety

- Test anxiety can be a formidable adversary. We'll provide tips and techniques for keeping anxiety under control on test day.

- Discover relaxation exercises and mindfulness strategies to maintain a calm and focused mindset.

Staying Flexible

- Sometimes, despite your best efforts, things don't go as planned on test day. Learn how to stay flexible and adapt to unexpected challenges, ensuring they don't derail your performance.

Post-Test Strategies

- What you do after the DAT Exam can also impact your overall performance. We'll provide guidance on reviewing your test experience and what steps to take next.

Test-Taking Ethics

- Understand the importance of maintaining test-taking ethics and the consequences of dishonest behavior during the DAT Exam.

Practice and Mock Tests

- The more you practice, the more confident you'll become. Explore the value of taking practice and mock tests and how they can sharpen your skills and strategies.

This chapter equips you with the tools needed to excel on test day, from effective strategies for tackling questions to techniques for managing test anxiety. With the right approach and preparation, you'll be ready to conquer the DAT Exam and take a significant step toward achieving your dream of becoming a dentist.

ADDITIONAL RESOURCES

In your quest to excel in the Dental Admission Test (DAT) Exam, it's essential to have a wide range of resources at your disposal. This chapter is dedicated to providing you with a comprehensive list of recommended online resources and academic materials to enhance your DAT preparation.

Recommended Online Resources

- Online resources are a valuable addition to your study plan. We've curated a list of websites, forums, and platforms that offer DAT-related content and support.

- Explore these online resources for additional practice questions, study aids, and forums for connecting with fellow DAT aspirants.

Recommended Academic Materials

- In addition to online resources, academic materials can provide in-depth coverage of DAT topics. We've gathered a list of recommended textbooks, study guides, and reference materials to supplement your study plan.

- Find out where to access academic materials that delve into the specific subjects covered in the DAT Exam, including biology, chemistry, and mathematics.

DAT Practice Tests and Simulations

- Practice makes perfect. Discover the importance of taking DAT practice tests and simulations and where to find them.

- Access valuable practice exams that mimic the DAT Exam's format and difficulty level, allowing you to gauge your readiness and improve your test-taking skills.

Tutoring and Review Courses

- For those seeking personalized guidance, we'll explore the benefits of DAT tutoring and review courses.

- Learn about the advantages of one-on-one tutoring or enrolling in comprehensive review courses to receive expert guidance and instruction.

Anki Decks and Flashcards

- Flashcards can be a powerful memorization tool. We'll introduce Anki decks and flashcards specifically designed for DAT preparation.

- Find out how to use these resources to reinforce your knowledge of key DAT concepts and terminology.

DAT Study Apps

- In today's digital age, study apps offer convenience and flexibility. We'll showcase DAT study apps that can help you prepare on the go.

- Explore mobile apps that provide interactive practice questions and other study materials.

DAT Study Groups and Communities

- Connecting with other DAT aspirants can provide support and motivation. We'll introduce DAT study groups and communities where you can engage with like-minded individuals.

- Discover the benefits of collaborative learning and sharing experiences with your peers.

Official ADA Resources

- The American Dental Association (ADA) offers official DAT resources. We'll guide you on how to access and utilize these authoritative materials.

- Explore ADA's DAT publications and practice exams, which can closely align with the actual DAT Exam.

Research Journals and Scientific Publications

- For those looking to delve deeper into DAT subjects, we'll suggest research journals and scientific publications.

- Find out where to access academic literature that can provide comprehensive insights into topics covered in the DAT Exam.

Dental School Admission Resources

- Preparing for the DAT Exam is just one part of your journey to dental school. We'll provide information on resources related to the dental school admission process.

- Learn about tools and guides that can assist you in crafting your dental school application and preparing for interviews.

This chapter serves as a valuable directory of resources to complement your DAT preparation. With access to these recommended materials, you'll have a well-rounded approach to mastering the DAT Exam and pursuing your dream of a successful dental career.

FINAL WORDS

As you reach the conclusion of your journey through the pages of this book, it's essential to reflect on the incredible commitment and effort you've invested in preparing for the Dental Admission Test (DAT) Exam. This final chapter is designed to provide you with words of encouragement and motivation, reminding you of the extraordinary potential within you and the boundless opportunities that await.

The Power of Persistence

- Success in the DAT Exam, and in life, often comes to those who persevere. Remember that persistence is a powerful force, and every moment of study brings you closer to your goals.

- Embrace the challenges, setbacks, and uncertainties as part of your growth journey. It's these experiences that shape your character and resilience.

Embracing Resilience

- Resilience is the ability to bounce back from adversity. Throughout your DAT preparation, you've undoubtedly faced hurdles and moments of doubt.

- Embrace these challenges as opportunities for growth. Every question you couldn't answer and every tough practice test were building your strength and knowledge.

Celebrating Progress

- Take time to acknowledge and celebrate your achievements, no matter how small they may seem. Completing a chapter, mastering a complex concept, or achieving a higher practice test score—all of these are milestones on your journey to success.

- Recognize that progress is not always linear, and success comes to those who persist and improve continuously.

Overcoming Self-Doubt

- Self-doubt can be a formidable opponent, but remember that you have come this far because you believe in your potential.

- Embrace your doubts as a sign that you are pushing your boundaries and aspiring for greatness. In the face of uncertainty, you have the power to prove yourself wrong.

Building Confidence

- Confidence is not something you either have or don't have—it can be developed and nurtured. Continue to build your confidence through consistent study and preparation.

- Trust in your abilities and the resilience you've developed along this journey. You are well-prepared to face the DAT Exam with courage.

Your Journey Beyond the DAT

- The DAT Exam is a stepping stone to a more profound journey—the pursuit of your dreams and a future in the field of dentistry.

- Keep your long-term goals in sight, knowing that the DAT is just one chapter in your extraordinary story.

Making a Difference

- As you move forward in your dental career, remember the impact you can have on the lives of others. Dentists make a difference in the health and well-being of their patients every day.

- Your dedication to the DAT Exam is a testament to your commitment to making a positive impact in the world.

Your Unseen Potential

- It's easy to underestimate your own potential. Yet, the determination and passion that have brought you this far are a testament to the extraordinary possibilities within you.

- Trust in your unseen potential to achieve greatness in the DAT Exam and your future career.

This final chapter is not an end but a beginning—a reminder that your journey is one of boundless potential and endless opportunities. Embrace every challenge and uncertainty as part of your growth, and let your preparation for the DAT Exam be a stepping stone to your dreams of becoming a dentist.

Your story is unique and extraordinary, and we have every confidence that you are destined for success. The DAT Exam is the gateway to your future, and you are well-equipped to walk through it with confidence and determination.

EXPLORE OUR RANGE OF STUDY GUIDES

At Test Treasure Publication, we understand that academic success requires more than just raw intelligence or tireless effort—it requires targeted preparation. That's why we offer an extensive range of study guides, meticulously designed to help you excel in various exams across the USA.

Our Offerings

- **Medical Exams:** Conquer the MCAT, USMLE, and more with our comprehensive study guides, complete with practice questions and diagnostic tests.

- **Law Exams:** Get a leg up on the LSAT and bar exams with our tailored resources, offering theoretical insights and practical exercises.

- **Business and Management Tests:** Ace the GMAT and other business exams with our incisive guides, equipped with real-world examples and scenarios.

- **Engineering & Technical Exams:** Prep for the FE, PE, and other technical exams with our specialized guides, which delve into both fundamentals and complexities.

- **High School Exams:** Be it the SAT, ACT, or AP tests, our high school range is designed to give you a competitive edge.

- **State-Specific Exams:** Tailored resources to help you with exams unique to specific states, whether it's teacher qualification exams or state civil service exams.

Why Choose Test Treasure Publication?

- **Comprehensive Coverage:** Each guide covers all essential topics in detail.

- **Quality Material:** Crafted by experts in each field.

- **Interactive Tools:** Flashcards, online quizzes, and downloadable resources to complement your study.

- **Customizable Learning:** Personalize your prep journey by focusing on areas where you need the most help.

- **Community Support:** Access to online forums where you can discuss concerns, seek guidance, and share success stories.

Contact Us

For inquiries about our study guides, or to provide feedback, please email us at support@testtreasure.com.

Order Now

Ready to elevate your preparation to the next level? Visit our website www.testtreasure.com to browse our complete range of study guides and make your purchase.